# DO MENOPAUSE MAGNIFICENTLY
# THE BURKENSTOCK PROTOCOL

## *BECAUSE YOU ARE SO WORTH IT!*

# KELLY BURKENSTOCK, M.D.

## FOREWORD BY MARISA PEER

ISBN

978-1-7346866-2-3 (ebook)

978-1-7346866-3-0 (paperback)

978-1-7346866-4-7 (paperback color)

Disclaimer

This book is not intended as a substitute for the medical advice of physicians. The reader should regularly consult a physician in matters relating to their health, particularly with respect to any symptoms that may require diagnosis or medical attention.

Published by Platinum Media Solutions

Charlotte, NC

704 200-2239

PlatinumMediaSolutions.com.

# Table of Contents

# Dedication

To every woman navigating the seasons of change—May you embrace this chapter with grace, vitality, and confidence.

These can truly be the best years of your life—filled with renewed energy, deeper connection, and the most meaningful intimacy you've ever known.

To the colleagues and mentors who've shared their insights along the way—thank you for your support as I continue to lead the conversation and set the standard in women's sexual health.

With unwavering dedication,
Dr. Kelly Burkenstock

# Foreword

I first met Dr. Kelly Burkenstock in New York in 2022, as the world was emerging from the pandemic's shadow. She had enrolled in my Rapid Transformational Therapy (RTT) certification course, eager to deepen her skills in RTT hypnotherapy. We quickly formed a bond—two professionals passionate about transforming lives, sharing ideas, insights, and reflections on the pandemic's profound impact.

Our conversations naturally evolved into a shared fascination: the extraordinary plasticity of the brain and the power to create meaningful change in people's lives. Dr. Burkenstock's approach to anti-aging, menopause, and women's health is fresh, innovative, and deeply rooted in a holistic philosophy. Her wisdom on living one's best life at any age is inspiring, blending science, compassion, and a fierce commitment to empowering women.

Dr. Burkenstock has become more than a colleague—she is a trusted friend and collaborator. She has followed me through seminars and workshops across the United States, Spain, and Portugal, always eager to learn and expand her knowledge. Her dedication to helping women—through every stage of life, from fertility and PCOS to menopause and beyond—is unmatched.

With over 20 years of experience, Dr. Burkenstock has built an impressive career. She holds a fellowship in Anti-Aging Medicine, a medical doctorate (M.D.) from LSUMC, and a Master's in Business Administration (M.B.A.) from UNO. She serves as a board member for the national Menopause Association (menopauseassociation.org) and is a constituent of the International Society for Sexual Medicine (ISSM) and the Sexual Medicine Society of North America (SMSNA). She is devoted to improving the health and well-being of women.

Together, we've explored how Rapid Transformational Therapy (RTT), combined with her groundbreaking holistic, natural protocols, can create powerful, synergistic results for women facing a variety of challenges.

Dr. Burkenstock has an infectious smile, an indomitable spirit, and a heart that's fully invested in the well-being of her clients. When you meet her, you instantly know she's in your corner.

This book is a gift for women who want to understand how to thrive through the seasons of womanhood, especially during the remarkable chapters of menopause.

By incorporating Dr. Burkenstock's Protocol into your life, you'll discover that menopause isn't just an ending—it's an opportunity to step into a vibrant, healthy, and empowered new beginning. This is a must-read.

~Marisa Peer

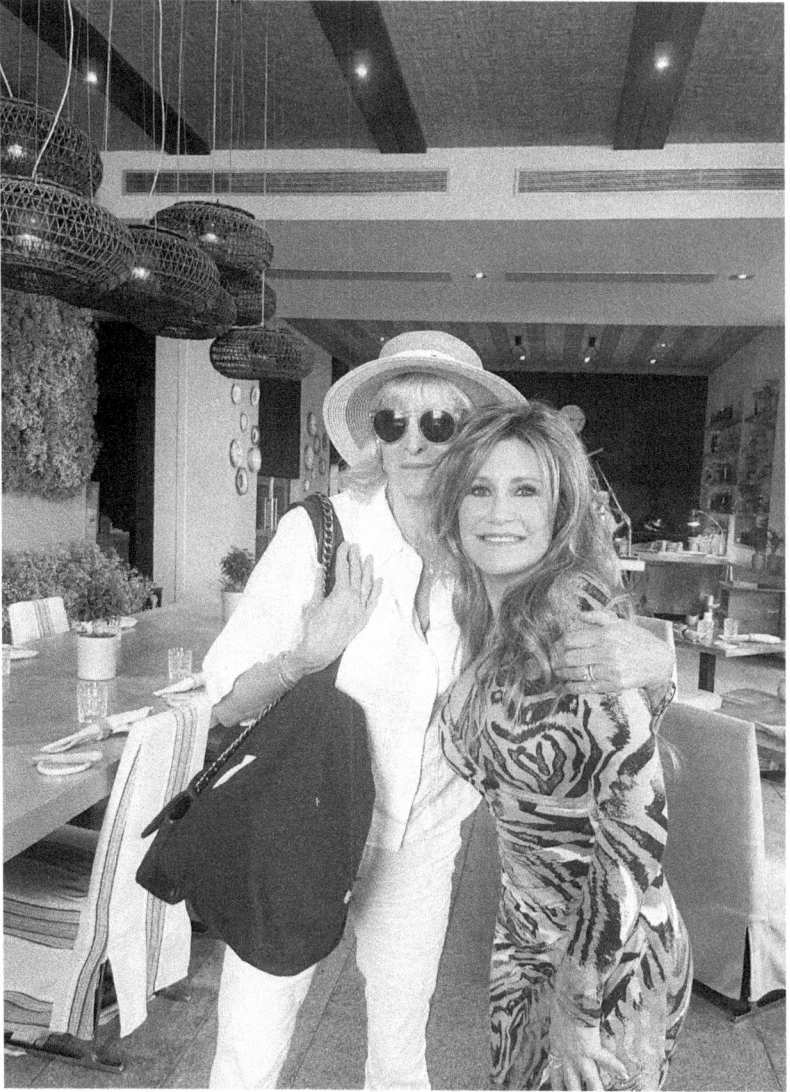

Marisa Peer & Dr. Burkenstock Douro, Portugal

# Introduction

Welcome to "Do Menopause Magnificently!" where you can age gracefully with the Burkenstock Protocol. I'm Dr. Kelly Burkenstock, and I'm thrilled to share my passion for women's health, especially concerning menopause and Anti-Aging. As a national speaker, educator, and recognized physician specializing in Anti-Aging and Regenerative medicine, I've dedicated my life to helping women feel fabulous and look fantastic at every stage of life.

As a young, green physician in 1999, I quickly learned that women after the age of 45 were suffering. Many were thrown on antidepressants and told their moodiness and brain fog were "all in their head." Frustrated with the lack of great options for ladies in western medicine, I began my studies abroad and earned a Fellowship in Anti-Aging and Regenerative Medicine—an Eastern medicine philosophy.

I became known as the Eastern-Western blend doctor, offering new solutions to empower women on their health and wellness journey.

In this book, we'll dive deep into the world of women's health, exploring everything from the science of menopause to cutting-edge treatments that can help you live your best life. We'll discuss hormones and genetics and how they impact your overall well-being. We'll explore innovative therapies like The O-Shot® Procedure and High-Intensity Focused Electromagnetic (HIFEM) Stimulation technology fields for enhancing sexual health and improving urinary incontinence, Platelet-Rich Plasma (PRP) for non-surgical facelifts, and personalized approaches to weight loss through DNA testing and food sensitivity identification.

But this isn't just about medical treatments; it's about embracing a holistic approach to health, menopause, and glamour. We'll discuss lifestyle factors, skincare regimens, and mindset practices that can help you age gracefully and confidently. I'll share my philosophy of integrating wellness and beauty, which I call the "Burkenstock Protocol."

Throughout this book, you'll find practical advice, actionable strategies, and the latest scientific insights to help you take control of your health and vitality. This book is for anyone approaching menopause, in the thick of it, or looking for ways to optimize their health post-menopause.

---

**─YOU ARE SO WORTH IT!...** ─────────────

Whether you are 40 and Fabulous, 50 and Fantastic, 60 and Sexy, 70 and Sensational, or Beyond, this is the time to live your best life! Join me, Dr. B., on this incredible journey.

---

# Part I

# Understanding
# Women's Health

# Chapter 1

# INTRODUCTION TO WOMEN'S HEALTH

When we talk about women's health, we're not just talking about reproductive issues or "female problems." We're talking about a complex, interconnected endocrine and biological network that affects every aspect of a woman's life. From hormones to heart health, bone density to brain function, female health is a rich and diverse field that deserves our full attention.

As women, our bodies go through many changes throughout our lives: puberty, pregnancy, perimenopause, menopause, and post-menopause. Each stage brings unique challenges and opportunities for growth and vitality. Understanding these changes is the first step in taking control of your health and well-being.

*Menopause* is one of the most significant transitions in a woman's life. It's a natural process, but it can feel anything but natural for many women. Hot flashes, mood swings, weight gain, skin changes, and sleep disturbances are just a few of the symptoms that can make this transition challenging. But ladies, take note, menopause doesn't have to be a negative experience! With proper knowledge and support, it can be a time of empowerment and renewal.

Hormones are powerful chemical messengers that are crucial to women's health. Estrogen, progesterone, testosterone (yes, women need testosterone, too!) and many other hormones work together in a delicate balance to regulate over 400 bodily functions. When this balance is disrupted during menopause, it can lead to a wide range of symptoms and health issues.

---

**A mature woman has earned wisdom.**
**She knows about life, her body, and her sexuality.**
**~Dr. Burkenstock**

---

However, hormones aren't the whole story. Genetics, lifestyle factors, and environmental influences all play a role in women's health. So, a holistic anti-aging approach that looks at the whole woman rather than treating individual problems or symptoms is essential.

In my practice, I've seen countless women transform their lives by taking charge of their health. It's not about turning back the clock or looking 20 years younger. It's about feeling phenomenal, looking magnificent, and living your marvelous life at any age because... *You Are So Worth It!*

I started seeing Dr. Burkenstock in 2006. The regimen she provided, hormones, supplements, and nutrition over the years has more than improved my overall well-being and anti-aging. From managing my weight, sleep, hair, skin, as well as moods, I gained back years of wellness. It's noticeable when people ask," What are you doing? I want what you have!" My answer is: "Go see Dr. B!"

*~RA Boudreaux*

In the following chapters, as we dive deeper into women's health, I want you to keep one thing in mind: Every woman is unique. Your body, genetics, and life experiences are all uniquely yours. So, your approach to health should be personalized, too. What works for your best friend or sister might not work for you, and that's okay.

We'll explore various treatments and therapies, from traditional to a more natural hormone replacement therapy to cutting-edge approaches like PRP and DNA testing for weight loss. We'll look at natural remedies, lifestyle changes, and mindset shifts that can make a life-changing difference for the rest of your long, gorgeous life.

I will show you how to advocate for yourself in your preventive healthcare journey. Too often, women's health concerns are dismissed; many times, they are given unnecessary prescriptions or not taken seriously.

*It's not all in your head*. I want to liberate you with the knowledge and confidence to speak up for yourself and get the care you deserve.

> Life is 10% what happens to you and 90% how you react.
>
> *~Charles R. Swindoll*

When I was delivering my youngest child at age 34, the OB-GYN tied my fallopian tubes as a method for future birth control. Tying the tubes does prevent pregnancy. However, after surgery, I immediately began experiencing insomnia. I inquired whether the tube-tying procedure could have affected my sleep.

The doctor answered, "No, my dear, you have three small children, and you are in medical school. You are just stressed." The science on insomnia secondary to the tubal ligation procedure had not yet been discovered. We now know that cutting a woman's fallopian tubes often interrupts the flow of progesterone, the *put-you-to-sleep* hormone. My new onset insomnia was due to my lack of progesterone and not my babies.

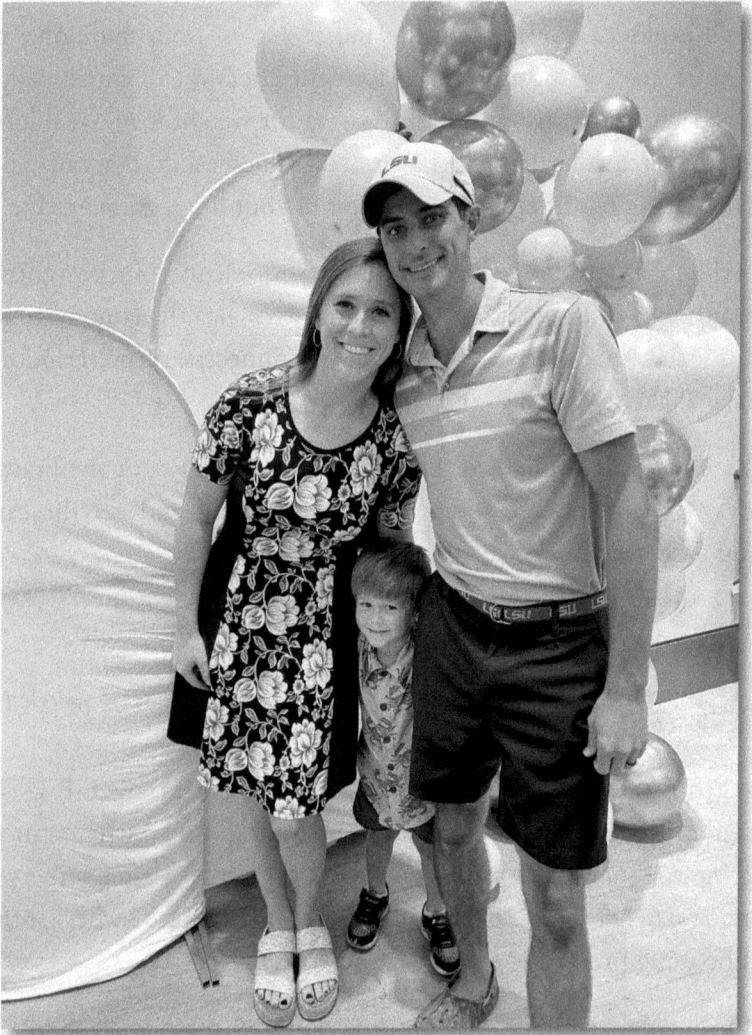

Chandler Burkenstock Hayes, Caspian & M.P. Hayes

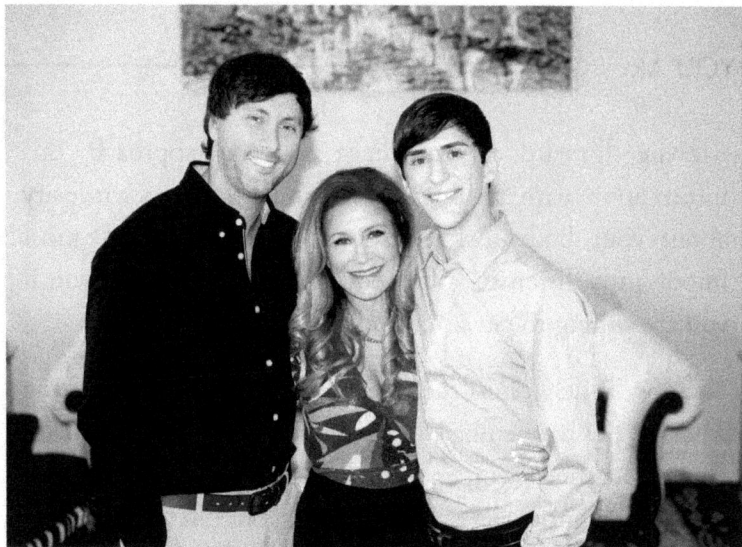

Dr. Austin, Dr. Kelly & Blaze Burkenstock, PA, PMC

Abstract[1]

Progesterone is present in many biological activities within a variety of tissues. This hormone affects reproduction, sleep quality, respiration, mood, appetite, learning, memory, and sexual activity. Progesterone exerts a sleep induction or hypnotic effect. It is a potent breathing or respiratory stimulant, and at proper levels, has been associated with a decrease in the number of obstructive sleep apnea episodes in men.

---

[1] Effects of progesterone on sleep: a possible pharmacological treatment for sleep-breathing disorders? M L Andersen 1, L R A Bittencourt, I B Antunes, S Tufik; Affiliations expand; PMID: 17168724; DOI: 10.2174/092986706779026200

## ┌─YOU ARE SO WORTH IT!... ──────

Moving forward, I encourage you to approach this information with an open mind and a sense of curiosity about your body. Ask questions, take notes, and, most importantly, listen to your body. It has much to tell you if you are willing to pay attention.

Next, we'll delve into the science of menopause, exploring what's really happening in your body during this transition and why it affects women in such different ways. We'll break down the complex hormonal changes and discuss how they affect various aspects of your health.

# *Chapter 2*

## THE SCIENCE OF MENOPAUSE

The science behind menopause is fascinating. Understanding what's happening in your body during this transition is key to navigating it successfully.

Menopause doesn't happen overnight; it's a gradual natural process that typically begins in your 40s or early 50s. This transition period, called perimenopause, can last anywhere from a few months to several years. Other women go through surgical menopause, where a partial or total hysterectomy is performed for medical reasons.

So, what's happening in your body during this time? It all comes down to hormones.

As you approach menopause, your ovaries start to produce less estrogen and progesterone. These hormones have been running the show in your body for decades, regulating your menstrual cycle. They support bone health, help maintain skin elasticity, and so much more.

> **Just as autumn prepares nature for winter, menopause prepares a woman's body for the post-reproductive years.**

The decrease in these hormones doesn't happen in a smooth, gradual way. Instead, levels can fluctuate wildly, so you might experience symptoms that come and go or vary in intensity. One day, you're fine; the next, you're a hot, sweaty mess!

Eventually, your ovaries stop releasing eggs, and your menstrual periods end. You've officially reached menopause when you've gone 12 consecutive months without a period. After that, you're considered in menopause or postmenopausal—the terms are interchangeable.

But here's the thing: menopause isn't just about reproductive function. These hormonal changes affect nearly every system in your body. That's why menopause can come with such a wide array of symptoms, from hot flashes to mood swings, high blood pressure, weight gain, and changes in skin and hair.

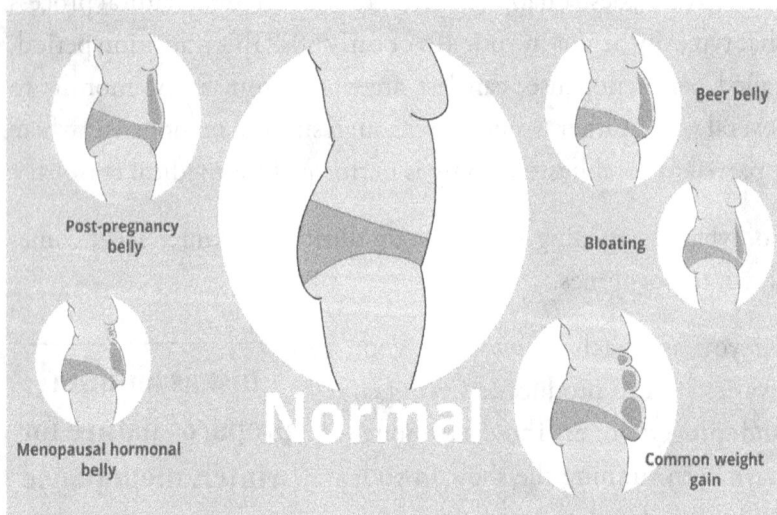

## SOME KEY PLAYERS IN THIS HORMONAL ORCHESTRA

### ESTROGEN

This isn't just one hormone but a group of hormones. The main ones are estrone (E1), estradiol (E2), and estriol (E3). Estradiol is the most active form during your reproductive years, but its levels drop significantly during menopause.

### PROGESTERONE

Progesterone is the major hormone for sleep quality. This hormone is crucial in preparing the uterus for pregnancy each month. When you are no longer producing eggs, progesterone levels plummet.

### TESTOSTERONE

Yes, women produce testosterone too! It's vital for libido, bone health, and muscle mass. Testosterone levels decline with age, but not as dramatically as estrogen and progesterone.

### FOLLICLE-STIMULATING HORMONE (FSH) AND LUTEINIZING HORMONE (LH)

As estrogen levels drop, your body produces more of these hormones to kick-start your ovaries. High levels of FSH and LH are often used to diagnose menopause. Understanding these hormonal changes can help explain why you might be experiencing specific symptoms. For example, decreasing estrogen levels can lead to bone loss, putting postmenopausal women at higher risk for osteoporosis. A drop in estrogen can also affect your skin's collagen production, leading to increased wrinkles and dryness.

## KEGEL EXERCISES

As women mature, many experience urinary leakage when laughing or coughing. This is due to pelvic floor muscle relaxation. More severe pelvic relaxation can lead to the uterus, bladder, urethra, or rectum protruding into the vagina. Kegel exercises are mandatory to keep the pelvic muscles strong. There are cutting-edge treatments we will discuss in future chapters to help with our all-important pelvic floor strength.

---

### YOU ARE SO WORTH IT!...

Menopause is a natural transition, not a disease. Yes, it can come with challenges, but it also marks the beginning of a new phase of life. Many women report feeling more confident, creative, and sexually free after menopause.

Keep reading to learn how these hormonal changes impact various aspects of your health and what you can do to support your body during this transition.

We'll also explore strategies for managing common menopause symptoms and discuss how proper hormone balance can help you feel your best.

---

God grant me the Serenity to accept the things I cannot change, the Courage to change the things I can, and the Wisdom to know the difference.

~Reinhold Niebuhr

# *Chapter 3*

## HORMONES AND THEIR IMPACT ON WOMEN'S HEALTH

Hormones are like the body's chemical messengers, coordinating complex processes like growth, metabolism, and fertility. When these messengers get out of sync, it can affect everything from your mood to your heart rhythm to your bones to your waistline.

Let's start by talking about two conditions that many women face: **Polycystic Ovary Syndrome (PCOS)** and **Premenstrual Syndrome (PMS)**. Both are closely tied to hormonal imbalances.

### POLYCYSTIC OVARY SYNDROME (PCOS)

PCOS is a common endocrine disorder that affects women of reproductive age. It's characterized by irregular periods, excess androgen (male hormones) levels, and often small cysts on the ovaries. Women with PCOS often struggle with issues like weight gain, acne, alopecia (hair loss), breast discharge, and fertility problems. The exact cause of PCOS isn't fully understood, but it involves a complex interplay of genetic and environmental factors.

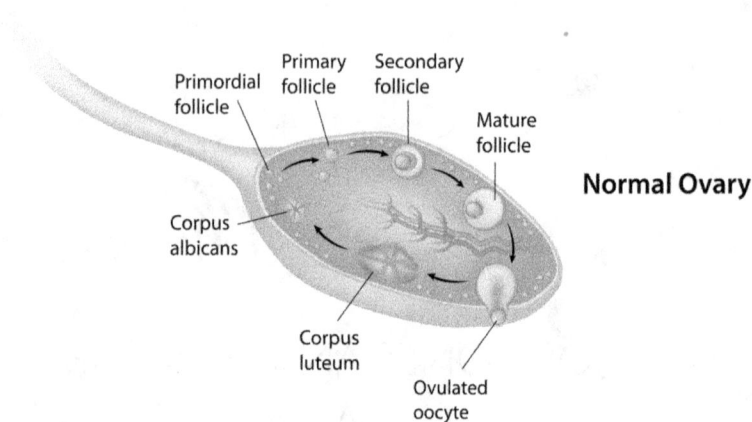

Normal Ovary

Primordial follicle
Primary follicle
Secondary follicle
Mature follicle
Corpus albicans
Corpus luteum
Ovulated oocyte

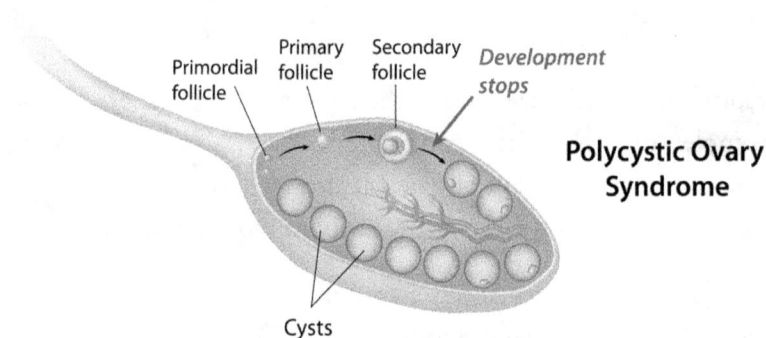

Polycystic Ovary Syndrome

Primordial follicle
Primary follicle
Secondary follicle
Development stops
Cysts

## MANAGING PCOS

Western medicine treats PCOS with prescriptions such as metformin, spironolactone, and birth control pills.

Eastern (alternative) medicine takes a better approach: a high-fiber/low-glycemic diet, Omega-3 fish oil, N-acetyl cysteine, Vitamin D, Synbiotics (prebiotics and probiotics), and exercise. A natural bioidentical hormone cream prescription may be considered only after implementing these natural Eastern therapies (i.e., holistic, alternative).

## PMS

PMS, on the other hand, is something that most women experience to some degree. The symptoms, which can include mood swings, bloating, cravings, cramps, breast tenderness, and more, are tied to the hormonal fluctuations of the menstrual cycle. These symptoms can be severe enough to interfere with daily life for some women.

## ESTRADIOL

Estradiol is the most potent and productive form of estrogen, and it plays a crucial role in many bodily functions. As estradiol levels drop during menopause, you might experience:

- Hot flashes and night sweats

- Vaginal dryness and discomfort

- Mood changes, including increased risk of depression and anxiety

- Changes in skin elasticity and hydration

- Decreased bone density

- Changes in body fat distribution

- Decreased sexual desire and orgasm

Estradiol (E2) is crucial in hundreds of important body functions from vaginal health to brain and heart health. A decline in E2 estrogen can result in substantial and various multiorgan deterioration if natural bioidentical hormones aren't replenished.

Estriol (E3) has positive effects on cholesterol, hot flashes, vaginal dryness, and fights urinary tract infections, and blocks the bad cancer-causing estrogen, Estrone (E1).

## ADRENAL FUNCTION

Another vital aspect of hormonal health is adrenal function. Your adrenal glands produce several essential hormones, including cortisol (the stress hormone) and Dehydroepiandrosterone (DHEA–a precursor to sex hormones). During menopause, your adrenal glands play a more significant role in hormone production.

Some women experience high adrenal function, leading to symptoms like anxiety, insomnia, and feeling "wired but tired." Others might have low adrenal function, resulting in fatigue, low blood pressure, and difficulty handling stress.

Proper supplementation can be extremely helpful in supporting adrenal function and overall hormonal balance. A supplement containing adrenal adaptogens is highly beneficial. If cortisol is high, the adrenal supplement adapts and helps pull it down to neutral. Also, if the cortisol plummets, the adrenal adaptogen helps raise it to neutral.

Adaptogens like Ashwagandha and Rhodiola, vitamins such as B2, B5, B6, Vitamin C, tyrosine, ginseng, and licorice support adrenal hormone balance; especially when used together, they have a synergistic effect.

Hormonal balance isn't just about estrogens and progesterone. It's a complex symphony of many different hormones, including thyroid hormones, testosterone, cortisol, insulin, and more. That's why it's so important to take a holistic approach to hormone health.

## HORMONE BALANCING

Balancing the Hormone symphony improves just about every aspect of your life. You experience an elevated mood, more energy, and a sharper mind. You will also find that you are sleeping better and experiencing less stress and anxiety.

Hormone balancing means feeling fabulous, improving vitality, and living longer!

**Dr. Burkenstock's Approach to Comprehensive Hormone Testing**

In my practice, I always start with comprehensive hormone testing to obtain a clear picture of what's going on in your body so we can create a personalized treatment plan.

Plans might include:

- Bioidentical hormone replacement therapy

- Dietary changes

- Targeted supplementation

- Stress management techniques.

Hormones should be tested by urine, saliva, or bloodwork every three to six months for proper monitoring and adjustments. You wouldn't close your eyes to drive; much the same, monitoring your hormone levels is essential.

—YOU ARE SO WORTH IT!...

As we wrap up this chapter, I want to emphasize that you don't have to live with hormonal imbalances. Whether you're dealing with PCOS, severe PMS, menopausal symptoms, or other hormonal issues, natural and prescription solutions are available. Finding what works best for you may take some time and experimentation, but don't give up. Your hormonal health greatly affects your overall well-being, and it's absolutely worth the effort to get it right.

Next, we'll examine the common symptoms and challenges of menopause, and I'll share some strategies for managing them effectively.

Ready to transform your life!
Scan or Call now to schedule a consult with Dr. Burkenstock

985-727-7676

# *Chapter 4*

## COMMON MENOPAUSE SYMPTOMS AND CHALLENGES

Every woman's menopause journey is unique, but there are some common symptoms and challenges that many of us face. Understanding these can help you feel more prepared and empowered to manage them effectively.

### SYMPTOMS OF MENOPAUSE

- Aching ankles, wrists, shoulders, heels

- Back pain

- Bloating

- Breast tenderness

- Decreased sexual interest

- Decreased ability to climax

- Depression

- Dizzy spells

- Facial hair growth
- Frequent urination
- Hair loss
- Hot flashes
- Insomnia
- Irritability
- Memory lapses/ decreased focus & concentration
- Migraine headaches
- Mood swings
- Night sweats
- Osteoporosis/osteopenia
- Painful intercourse
- Palpitations/ heart fluttering
- Panic attacks
- Reflux
- Skin feeling crawly
- Snoring
- Urinary leakage/incontinence
- Urinary tract infections
- Vaginal dryness
- Vaginal itching
- Vaginal odor
- Varicose veins/ spider veins
- Vivid dreams
- Weight gain (especially lower abdomen)

## THE MOST COMMON SYMPTOMS OF MENOPAUSE

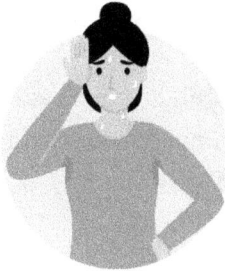

**HOT FLASHES** are probably the most well-known symptoms of menopause. That sudden feeling of heat spreading through your body, often followed by sweating and chills. They can be uncomfortable and disruptive.

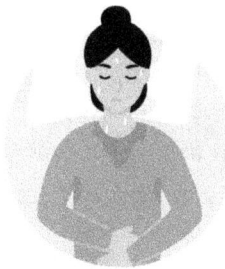

**NIGHT SWEATS** can severely impact your sleep quality, leading to fatigue and irritability.

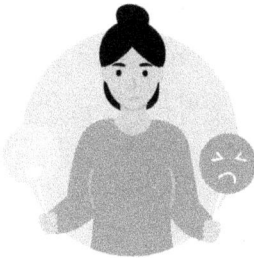

**MOOD CHANGES.** Don't be surprised if you find yourself on an emotional rollercoaster. Irritability, anxiety, and even depression are common during menopause. These mood swings aren't just "in your head". They're a real result of hormonal fluctuations.

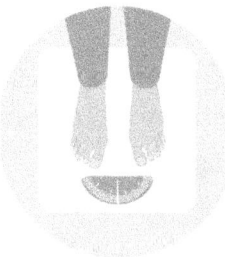

**WEIGHT GAIN AND CHANGES IN BODY COMPOSITION.** Many women notice weight gain, especially around the midsection (belly fat). As your metabolism slows down during menopause, your body tends to store fat differently and burn fat less efficiently.

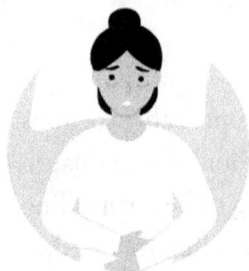

**SLEEP DISTURBANCES** like night sweats, anxiety, and a lack of progesterone (the sleep hormone), can make getting a good night's rest a real challenge. This can impact your energy levels, mood, and overall health.

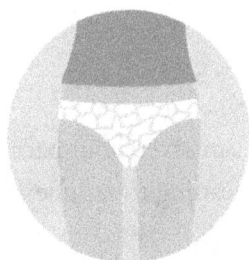

**VAGINAL DRYNESS AND DISCOMFORT.** As estrogen levels (E2, E3) drop, vaginal tissues can become thinner and less lubricated, which leads to discomfort during intercourse and increases the risk of urinary tract infections.

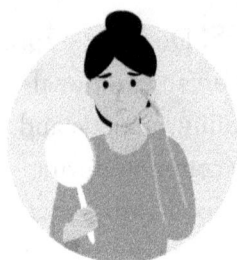

**HAIR THINNING OR LOSS, DRY SKIN.** You might notice your skin becoming drier and less elastic due to decreasing estrogen and collagen production. Many women's skin becomes creepy and thin.

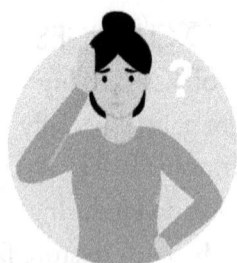

**BRAIN FOG.** Numerous women report difficulty concentrating or minor memory lapses during menopause.

"Our research team demonstrated that estradiol directly relates to changes in memory performance and reorganization of our brain circuitry that regulates memory function. Thus, women and men undergo different aging processes, especially in early midlife when reproductive aging is more critical for women than chronological aging."

~*Jill M. Goldstein, PhD, Harvard Medical School*

The work of Dr. Goldstein and others further emphasizes my plight to educate women about the importance and urgency of natural bioidentical hormone replacement therapy, especially as it relates to memory loss and Alzheimer's.

## MANAGING THE SYMPTOMS OF MENOPAUSE

Although this might seem daunting, not every woman experiences all these symptoms, and there are effective ways to manage them. In my practice, I've seen women overcome these challenges and thrive during menopause.

Effective strategies for managing menopause symptoms include:

- **Hormone Replacement Therapy (HRT)**: HRT can be very effective for managing many menopause symptoms. We'll dive deeper into HRT options in Chapter 7.

- **Lifestyle Changes**: Regular exercise, a healthy diet, and stress management techniques like meditation can be beneficial in symptom relief.

- **Targeted Supplements**: Specific vitamins, minerals, and herbs can help support your body during this transition. Targeted bloodwork to identify vitamin and mineral deficiencies can help to guide proper supplementation.

- **Vaginal Moisturizers and Lubricants**: These can help with vaginal dryness and discomfort. I recommend natural lubricants like virgin coconut oil.

- **Sleep Hygiene**: Establishing good sleep habits can help combat insomnia and fatigue. Remember, a cold, dark, and quiet bedroom enhances quality sleep.

- **Cognitive Behavioral Therapy**: This can help manage mood changes and anxiety.

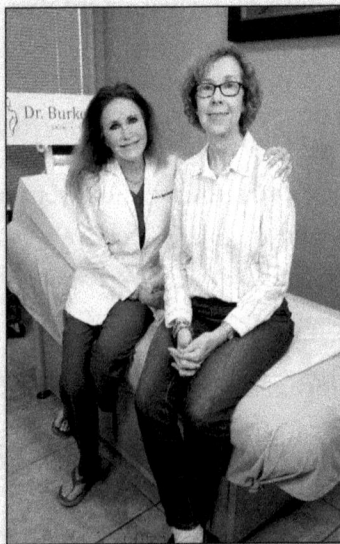

"I started Bioidentical hormones at 65 years old with Dr. Burkenstock, and I am thinking clearer, feel stronger, and look younger. The overall health benefits are definitely worth initiating hormones, even though I am not sexually active."

*~Mary P.*

## YOU ARE SO WORTH IT!...

Women's issues like PMS, Infertility, PCOS and Menopause are all common and treatable female issues. Menopause is a natural transition, not a disease. With the proper support and strategies, you can navigate these issues of life with grace and vitality. Don't hesitate to reach out to your Anti-aging physician or primary care if you're struggling with menopause symptoms. Don't suffer in silence. Menopause and beyond can be the best time of your long, gorgeous life!

The topic of our next chapter is often overlooked but incredibly important: **Sexual health during menopause**. We'll discuss how menopause can impact your sex life and what you can do to maintain a fulfilling and enjoyable intimate relationship.

Menopause is the beautiful dawn of a new chapter in a woman's life. She has gained so much wisdom and can finally prioritize her own happiness!

~Dr. Burkenstock

Ready to transform your life!
Scan or Call now to schedule a consult with Dr. Burkenstock

985-727-7676

# *Chapter 5*

## SEXUAL HEALTH AND MENOPAUSE

> "And the beauty of a woman, with passing years only grows!"
>
> ~*Audrey Hepburn*

### LET'S TALK ABOUT SEX, BABY!

I know, I know… it might feel a bit uncomfortable, but intimacy is an integral part of overall well-being, especially during and after menopause. Too often, women suffer in silence, thinking that a decline in sexual function is just something they must accept. But *Ladies, listen up... that is not true!*

Menopause can indeed bring changes to your sex life, but with the proper knowledge and tools, you can maintain—and even *improve*—your sex life and satisfaction.

Many reasons—from medications to past sexual trauma to health conditions—can make it difficult for some females to enjoy sex or achieve orgasm. Worry not if this applies to you; there's nothing wrong with you. You can still enjoy touch and pleasure even if you don't climax.

The clitoris is the primary organ of the female genitals responsible for pleasure. Did you know that your clitoris is not just the tiny button on the outside of your genital area? In fact, it is more like a bird with wings that extends upward and inside the vagina, and it has over 12,000 nerve endings. The clitoris develops from the same structure in the human embryo as the penis and is similarly sensitive to touch and arousal. It plays a key role in sexual stimulation and orgasm. With stimulation to the female genitals, the vagina widens and lengthens, preparing to accept the penis. For a woman, it usually takes 20 minutes for full sexual arousal, so relax, be patient, let the taboo go, and enjoy your journey. It's never too late to learn!

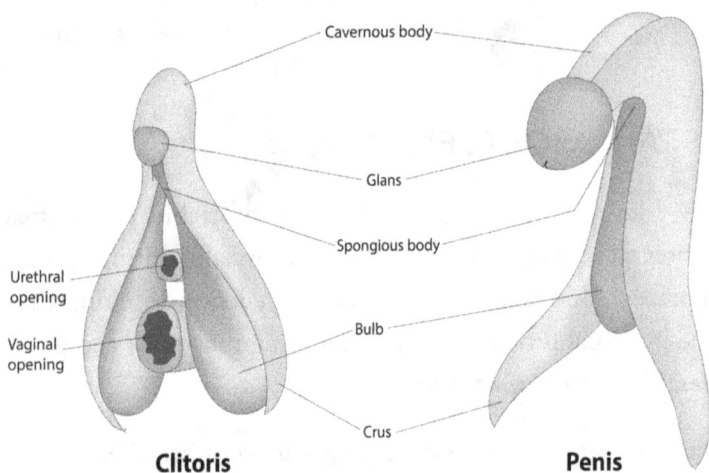

**Clitoris**  **Penis**

With knowledge and practice, you can get to know your body through self-touch, which can be a beautiful and healing experience. Also, you can get a vibrator and explore your magnificent body.

Many clients report a decrease in arousal as they age. For this, I prescribe our topical custom Arousal Scream Cream, intended to increase arousal, stimulation, and sexual satisfaction by increasing blood flow to the genitals. The cream is applied directly to the clitoris, vagina, and perineum 30 minutes before relations.

Did you know that an orgasm decreases infections, depression and aging? In fact, orgasms are Antiaging!

Let's chat about Multiple Orgasms! With a bit of knowledge and practice, they are attainable and fun. Orgasms produce *oxytocin* and other hormones, which are **Anti-aging!** Vaginas are uniquely suited to climaxing more than once, while penises tend to have a "refractory period" (time necessary between orgasms) to climax or ejaculate a second time.

> "Because there is more surface area on your vulva and inside your vagina, there's more ability for multiple orgasms. Once the first orgasm is enjoyed, switching up the pressure and exact location [of stimulation] can allow for more orgasms to follow."

Back to oxytocin. In a study (see below)[1], oxytocin was observed to have an Anti-aging effect on skin cells, possibly attributed to increased levels of the antioxidant glutathione (GSH). The 'in-love skin glow look' isn't just a romantic idea; it's a science-supported reality.

A compounding pharmacist can make oxytocin as a nasal spray, oral solution, or lozenge. It can also be increased *Naturally* by spending time with animals. Petting animals boosts oxytocin, lowers stress cortisol, and keeps blood pressure at bay.

---

[1] *Dermatology Times*, Feb 26, 2021, by Cheryl G. Krader, BS, Pharm, Clinical Study Points to Oxytocin's Antiaging Benefits. (https://www.dermatologytimes.com/view/clinical-study-points-to-oxytocin-s-antiaging-benefits)

UC Berkeley researchers (2024) have also discovered that oxytocin is indispensable for healthy muscle maintenance and repair. This hormone also helps prevent osteoporosis and, as a bonus, fights obesity. Oxytocin is the first Anti-aging molecule approved by the Food and Drug Administration for clinical use in humans. Clinical trials of oxytocin nasal spray are underway to alleviate symptoms associated with mental disorders such as autism, schizophrenia, and dementia.[2]

## SOLUTIONS FOR MENOPAUSE SYMPTOMS

### VAGINAL DRYNESS

Vaginal dryness is one of the most common complaints I hear from my menopausal patients. As estrogen levels drop, the vaginal tissues can become thinner and less lubricated. This can lead to discomfort or pain during intercourse.

**Solution**: My best recommendation is Virgin Coconut Oil. The oil's pH blends well with the vaginal tissue. It is silky, smells nice, and tastes pleasant. In a pinch, olive oil works well too. Water-based lubricants can be used, although they can be sticky, and the pH may *aggravate* the vagina, causing irritation. There are also vaginal moisturizers that can be used regularly to improve overall vaginal health. Topical estriol E3 creams or suppositories are recommended in many cases.

---

[2] https: Neural Regen Res. 2021 Dec; 16(12): 2413–2414.; Published online 2021 Apr 23. doi: 10.4103/1673-5374.313030; PMCID: PMC8374585; PMID: 33907023; The antiaging role of oxytocin; Tarek Benameur,# Maria A. Panaro,# and Chiara Porro, PhD; //www.ncbi.nlm.nih.gov/pmc/issues/388300/

## DECREASED LIBIDO

During menopause, many women notice a decrease in their sex drive. This can be due to hormonal changes and other factors like fatigue or mood changes.

**Solution**: Addressing overall hormone balance can help. We also look at testosterone levels, as this hormone plays a role in libido for women, too. Lifestyle factors like stress management and regular exercise can also boost libido. We offer several treatment options to restore the integrity and lubrication of the vaginal canal: High Frequency Electromagnetic Stimulation therapy, Platelet-rich plasma injections (PRP), otherwise known as The O-Shot® Procedure, Exosome stem cell injections, and the Red LED Personal Vaginal Wand.

## CHANGES IN SEXUAL RESPONSE

You might notice it takes longer to become aroused or to reach orgasm. This is normal and doesn't mean anything is the matter with you. Ladies, your wisdom, patience, and experience will help you overcome this tiny setback. Instead of running for a five-minute Intimacy session, a mature woman lingers for a more extended, meaningful experience. It takes time to build up the excitement- *Savor It!* And yes, *It Is So Worth It!*

**Solution**: Patience and communication with your partner are key. You may need to experiment with different types of stimulation or try new things to discover what works for you now. Adult toy shops or FUN shopping can be fun and intriguing—explore, try, experiment, and, by all means, ENJOY!

When we live in a world of shame and taboo, we may miss out on deep intimacy. You may want to explore Zenhabits.net, a website focused on *Mindfully Letting Go of Shame*.

## URINARY INCONTINENCE

Many women don't realize that urinary incontinence is connected to sexual health. Urinary leakage becomes more common after menopause and/or multiple childbirths, and incontinence can significantly impact your quality of life, including your sex life. Several of my mature female clients report leaking on couches and beds and suffer embarrassment. They also mention wearing diapers and are personally scorned with humiliation.

**Solution**: The fabulous news is that there's a lot you can do to address incontinence and improve your pelvic floor strength. Kegel exercises are a great place to start. These exercises strengthen the pelvic floor muscles, which support the bladder, uterus, and other pelvic organs.

Here's how to do a proper Kegel:

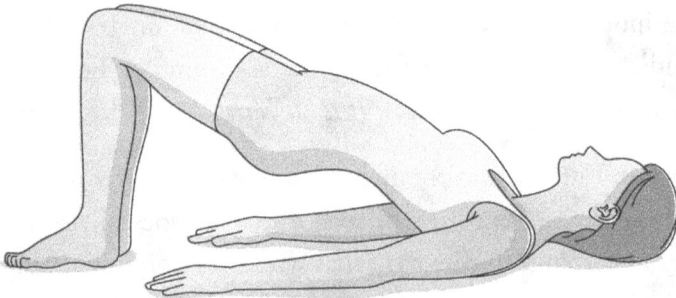

1. Identify the correct muscles by stopping urination midstream. The muscles that allow you to stop the stream are your pelvic floor muscles.

2. Tighten these muscles and hold for 5 seconds, then relax for 5 seconds. Think of an elevator's operation—pull the muscles in and up—this is a proper Kegel.

3. Repeat this 10 times, 3 times a day.

As the muscles get stronger, you can increase the duration of the hold and the number of repetitions.

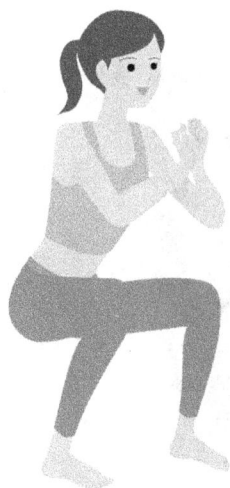

Squats are another excellent exercise for pelvic floor strengthening because they engage the core and the muscles around the pelvis. They also can help improve mobility and strengthen joints and bones.

*Bonus*: Strengthening your pelvic floor doesn't just help with incontinence; it can also increase sexual pleasure! Stronger pelvic floor muscles can lead to more intense orgasms and increased sensation during intercourse.

There are also advanced treatments available for both sexual health and incontinence. We have seen great results with several modalities:

**The O-Shot® Procedure:** This treatment uses platelet-rich plasma (PRP) and Exosomes to stimulate tissue regeneration in the vaginal and clitoral areas improving sexual function and reducing incontinence.

**HIFEM**: High Frequency Electromagnetic stimulation therapy is another cutting-edge treatment for pelvic floor dysfunction.

**Vaginal Wand:** After initial improvement with these treatments, we offer our clients a personal vaginal LED wand for home use which offers a combination of Red LED light, heat, and vibration to continue rejuvenation at home. We'll discuss these procedure options in more detail in a later chapter.

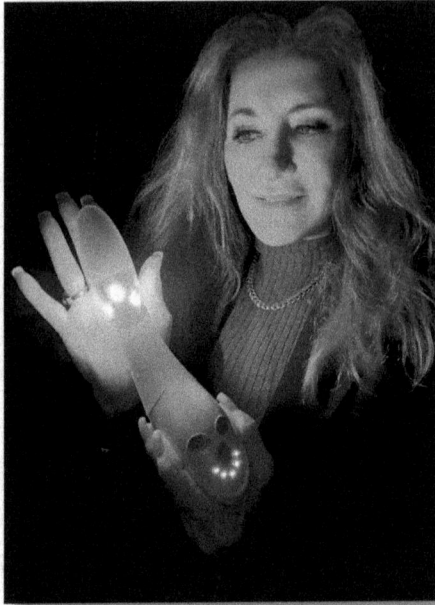

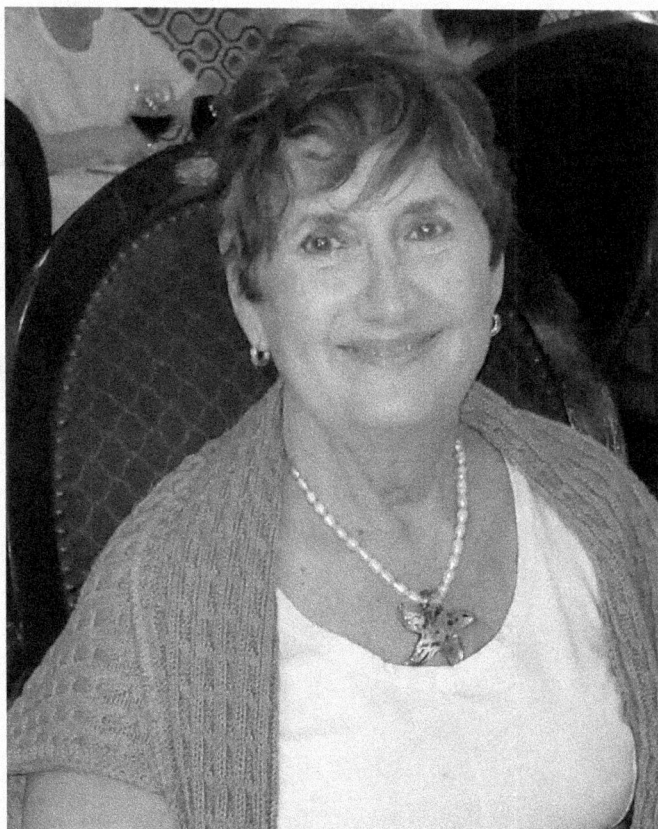

I have a pacemaker, so I was not a candidate for the HIFEM magnetic stimulation chair. I have been using the vaginal LED wand, and my urinary incontinence symptoms are Dramatically better! Thank you, Dr. Burkenstock.

~Marylyn R.

## YOU ARE SO WORTH IT!...

Sexual health is vital to your overall health and well-being. Don't be embarrassed to discuss concerns with your healthcare provider. We're here to help you live your best life, and that includes having a satisfying sex life.

In the next chapter, we'll uncover the role of genetics in women's health.

# *Chapter 6*

## THE ROLE OF GENETICS
## IN WOMEN'S HEALTH

You have probably heard the phrase, "It's in your genes," and there is much truth to this regarding health. Your genetic makeup can *influence*, but not determine, your destiny. Genes *influence* everything from your risk of certain diseases to how you respond to different foods and medications. Lifestyle choices and environment directly determine what actually presents in life.

Your genes are like a blueprint for your body, containing instructions for building and maintaining your cells. You inherit these genes from your parents, so family history is considered when assessing health risks. We can turn specific genes on or off through epigenetics and neuroplasticity. How we eat, exercise, and live helps our bodies decide which genes ultimately emerge in our lifetime.

> "The moment you change your perception, is the moment you rewrite the chemistry of your body."
>
> ~Dr. Bruce Lipton[1]

Genetics play a role in several areas of women's health:

## BREAST AND OVARIAN CANCER

Specific genetic mutations, like those in the BRCA1 and BRCA2 genes, can increase a woman's risk of developing breast and ovarian cancer. Genetic testing might be recommended if you have a strong family history of these cancers.

## OSTEOPOROSIS

Your genes can influence your bone density and how quickly you lose bone mass as you age. Some women are genetically predisposed to develop osteoporosis earlier than others. Eating well and exercising help downplay these genetic tendencies and prevent bone loss.

## HEART DISEASE

While lifestyle factors play a huge role in heart health, genetics can also impact your risk of heart disease. Your genes can influence factors like cholesterol levels and blood pressure. Have your physician run bloodwork, cardiac and carotid ultrasounds to be proactive in your heart health. Also, following Heart Rate Variability (HRV) helps monitor the body's homeostasis, which fights off disease development.

---

[1] Integr Med (Encinitas). 2017 Dec; 16(6):44-50. Bruce Lipton, PhD: *The Jump From Cell Culture to Consciousness.*

## AUTOIMMUNE DISEASES

Many autoimmune diseases, such as Lupus and Rheumatoid Arthritis, are more common in women and have a genetic component. Low dose naltrexone (LDN)[2] is an anti-aging prescription that has been used to treat symptoms of autoimmune diseases, cancer, and other conditions.

We'll talk more about LDN in Chapter 14.

## MENOPAUSE SYMPTOMS

Believe it or not, even your menopause experience can be influenced by your genes. The age at which you enter menopause and the severity of your symptoms can be partially determined by your genetic makeup. You might think, "If it's all in my genes, what can I do?" This is where the exciting field of epigenetics comes in. Epigenetics refers to changes in gene expression that do not involve changes to the underlying DNA sequence. In other words, while you can't change your genes, you can influence how they're expressed through lifestyle factors like diet, exercise, and stress management.

This is incredibly empowering because it means that even if you have a genetic predisposition to particular health issues, you're not doomed to develop them. Your lifestyle choices can have a significant impact on your health outcomes.

---

[2]Mediterr J Rheumatol. 2023 Mar 31;34(1):1-6. *Low-Dose Naltrexone in Rheumatological Diseases.* Jozelio Freire de Carvalho.

## WAYS YOU CAN USE THIS KNOWLEDGE TO YOUR ADVANTAGE:

### GENETIC TESTING

Consider genetic testing to understand your risk factors. This can help you and your healthcare physician develop a personalized prevention and screening plan.

### FAMILY HISTORY

Keep a detailed record of your family's health history. This can provide valuable insights into your genetic risks.

### PERSONALIZED NUTRITION

Your genetic makeup can influence how your body processes different nutrients. Nutrigenomics, the study of how genes and nutrients interact, can help you develop a diet plan tailored to your genetic profile. My clinics run a DNA guided Nutrigenomic report that shows how you should eat, exercise, and what brain mutations you have so we can build each client a custom lifestyle plan based on your genes. You may be built for a low-protein, high-carbohydrate, or even high-fat diet depending on your genes.

Read more about personalized nutrition in *Chapter 9 – Dare To Be Thin® DNA Testing for Weight Loss: Personalized Approaches to Optimal Weight.*

---

**Dare to Be Thin® The Answer is in your Genes!**
~ Dr. Burkenstock.

---

## EXERCISE

While exercise benefits everyone, certain types might be more effective based on your genetic makeup. Again, depending on whether you are built with fast twitch, slow twitch, or a combination of 50% fast/50% slow twitch muscle fiber types determines which exercises are most efficient in burning fat.

## STRESS MANAGEMENT

Your genes can influence how you respond to stress. Understanding this can help you develop more effective stress management strategies. I've seen remarkable results when we tailor treatment plans to a client's genetic profile. For example, we might adjust Hormone Replacement Therapy (HRT) based on how a woman's body metabolizes different hormones or recommend specific supplements based on genetic markers for nutrient absorption.

One exciting area of genetic research in women's health is pharmacogenomics—the study of how genes affect a person's response to drugs. This field holds great promise for personalizing medication choices and dosages, potentially improving efficacy and reducing side effects.

Remember, your genes are not your destiny. They're more like a roadmap, showing you areas where you might need to pay extra attention or take preventive action.

In the next chapter, we'll shift gears and explore various treatments and therapies for menopause and women's health issues. We'll begin with an overview of menopause treatments, from traditional hormone replacement therapy to alternative approaches.

Ready to transform your life!
Scan or Call now to schedule a consult with Dr. Burkenstock

985-727-7676

# Part II:
# Treatments and Therapies

Beginning in 2025, the FDA plans to remove the black box warning from Hormone Replacement Therapy (HRT), citing updated scientific evidence.

The decision aims to improve access to HRT by removing warnings about cardiovascular disease, breast cancer, and dementia..

# *Chapter 7*

## MENOPAUSE TREATMENTS

### FROM HORMONE REPLACEMENT THERAPY (HRT) TO ALTERNATIVE APPROACHES

Welcome to Part II of our journey! In Part I, we laid the groundwork for understanding women's health and menopause. So, let's dive into the various treatments and therapies available, from traditional hormone replacement therapy to alternative and complementary approaches.

We'll start with Hormone Replacement Therapy (HRT), which has been a game-changer for many women dealing with menopause symptoms. HRT involves supplementing your body with hormones no longer produced in sufficient quantities. Typically, this means estrogen (E2, E3) and progesterone, but also testosterone, DHEA, pregnenolone, and melatonin.

### TWO MAIN TYPES OF HRT

1. **Systemic hormone therapy** includes pills, patches, pellets, creams, gels, or sprays that release hormones into the bloodstream.

2. **Low-dose vaginal products** are used locally to treat vaginal and urinary symptoms.

In my clinics, we preferentially prescribe Bioidentical Natural Hormone Creams. These creams give the body an ongoing (even daily) dose of hormones. Since creams are external, we are not exposing our organs to hormones.

Many women and healthcare professionals still worry about the perceived risks of hormone replacement therapy (HRT). Much of the negativity regarding HRT stems from the misinterpretation of the Women's Health Initiative (WHI) study in 2002, which led to a worldwide reduction in HRT use. The subsequent sub-analysis of this study revealed that it had some significant flaws. When the data was re-examined, the findings actually supported the use of hormone therapy, especially in younger women. Other research has supported the National Institute for Health and Care Excellence menopause guidelines that state the benefits of HRT outweigh the risks in most women.

The Menopause Association position statement of 2022 confirms that hormone therapy remains the most effective treatment for menopausal symptoms. Also, for select survivors of breast and endometrial cancer, data shows that the use of low-dose vaginal estrogen therapy appears safe and greatly improves quality of life. (www.menopause.org)

The American Urological Association (AUA) has clearly communicated in the 2025 position statement that intravaginal estrogen and DHEA does Not cause breast or uterine or endometrial cancer and can be used in patients with a history of breast cancer under most situations.[1]

---

[1] Kaufman MR, Ackerman LA, Amin KA, et al. The AUA/SUFU/AUGS Guideline on Genitourinary Syndrome of Menopause. J Urol. 0(0).
doi:10.1097/JU.0000000000004589.
https://www.auajournals.org/doi/10.1097/JU.0000000000004589

Transdermal (topical on the skin) estrogen is the preferred route of administration because, in contrast with oral estrogen, estrogen as a patch or cream/gel is not associated with blood clots (venous thromboembolism). Most patches and gels are estradiol only, whereas, in our compounded creams, we combine Estradiol and Estriol, the two beneficial forms of Estrogen.

That being said, HRT isn't right for everyone. You should have a thorough discussion with your healthcare physician about your individual risks and benefits. Factors like your age, how long you've been in menopause, and your personal and family medical history all play a role in determining whether HRT is appropriate for you.

Dr. K. Holtorf, in his groundbreaking medical review,[2] states, "Physiological data and clinical outcomes demonstrate that bioidentical hormones are associated with lower risks, including the risk of breast cancer and cardiovascular disease, and are more efficacious than their synthetic and animal-derived counterparts. Until evidence is found to the contrary, bioidentical hormones remain the preferred method of hormone replacement therapy."

## THE BURKENSTOCK PROTOCOL

Now, let's talk about **bioidentical natural hormones**—hormones that are chemically identical to those your body produces. While there's still debate in the medical community about whether bioidentical hormones are safer or more effective than traditional HRT, my patients report feeling better and enjoying a better quality of life on bioidentical hormones. Many studies tout the safety profile of bioidentical HRT.

2 Holtorf, K., The bioidentical hormone debate: are bioidentical hormones (estradiol, estriol, and progesterone) safer or more efficacious than commonly used synthetic versions in hormone replacement therapy?" Postgrad Med 2009; 121 (1):73-85.

What if HRT isn't right for you, or you prefer to try other options first? There are several alternative approaches to managing menopause symptoms:

- **Phytoestrogens**: These are plant-based compounds that mimic estrogen in the body. They're found in fruits, vegetables, nuts and seeds, coffee, olive oil, and red wine. While the evidence is mixed, some women find relief from menopause symptoms by increasing their intake of phytoestrogens.

- **Herbal remedies**: Certain herbs, such as black cohosh, red clover, dong quai, evening primrose oil, and maca, have been traditionally used to manage menopause symptoms. While scientific evidence is mixed, many women report benefits from these herbs.

- **Acupuncture**: Some studies suggest that acupuncture may help with hot flashes, mood swings, insomnia, and other menopause symptoms.

- **Mind-body practices**: Techniques like Pilates, yoga, meditation, and tai chi can help manage stress and improve overall well-being during menopause.

- **Lifestyle modifications**: Never underestimate the power of a healthy diet, regular exercise, and good sleep habits in managing menopause symptoms.

*Note*: While soy does contain phytoestrogens, I do not recommend soy as it wreaks havoc on the thyroid and female hormones. It is a controversial food, with some studies showing it increases breast cancer risk.

One approach I've found particularly effective is combining bioidentical HRT with supplements, lifestyle, and dietary changes. This integrative approach allows us to address symptoms from multiple angles and often results in better outcomes.

It's also worth mentioning that there are non-hormonal prescription medications that help with specific menopause symptoms for women who are not candidates for HRT. Antidepressants (including paroxetine, venlafaxine, citalopram, and escitalopram), gabapentin, and sometimes low-dose clonidine can be used to help manage menopausal symptoms like hot flashes.

The key to successful menopause symptom treatment is personalization. What works wonderfully for your best friend might not be the right fit for you. Finding the right combination of treatments may take some trial and error.

In my med spas, I always start with a comprehensive evaluation, including testing for sex and thyroid hormones, and vitamin and mineral deficiencies. We then discuss our clients' symptoms and health history in detail. Based on this information, we can develop a tailored treatment plan that addresses their needs and concerns.

## YOU ARE SO WORTH IT!...

As we wrap up this chapter, I want to emphasize that menopause is not a one-size-fits-all experience, nor is its treatment. Communicate with your healthcare physician, and don't hesitate to explore different options.

Next, we'll learn about cutting-edge treatments for sexual health, low libido, and incontinence that are showing promising results. These innovative therapies are an example of how the field of women's health is evolving, offering new solutions for age-old problems.

The O-Shot® Procedure, the HIFEM (High Frequency Electromagnetic Stimulation therapy (for example, Emsella™), and the Vaginal Wand LED Stimulator (for example, Joylux™) are three new exciting breakthroughs for female sexual wellness and menopause. Keep reading for more details.

Ready to transform your life!
Scan or Call now to schedule a consult with Dr. Burkenstock

985-727-7676

# Chapter 8

## THE **OH LA LA!** TREATMENT PROTOCOLS ENHANCING SEXUAL HEALTH AND PLEASURE

Exciting and revolutionary treatments have arrived in women's Intimate health. These procedures are simple, hormone-free, pain-free, and do not require surgery. The "Orgasm PRP Shot" (O-Shot), the High Frequency Electromagnetic Stimulation Chair therapy (HIFEM), and the Red LED Personal Vaginal Wand (please contact us) have been game-changers for many of my clients to address issues like sexual dysfunction, vaginal dryness, decreased sensation, and urinary incontinence. So, what exactly are these innovative procedures, and how do they work?

The O-Shot® Procedure is a non-surgical procedure that uses your platelet-rich plasma (PRP) to rejuvenate and revitalize vaginal and clitoral tissue. PRP is derived from your blood, making it a natural and safe option for many women.

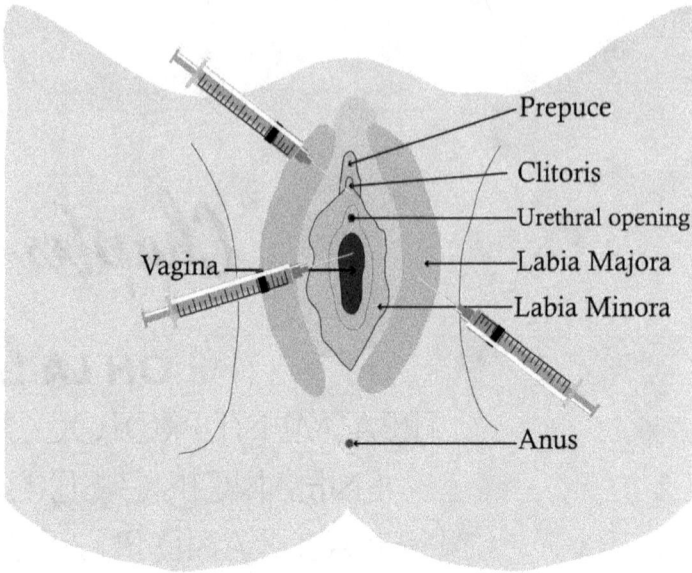

The O-Shot® Procedure works as follows:

1. A small amount of blood is drawn from your arm, just like a regular blood test.

2. The blood is then centrifuged to separate the platelet-rich plasma (PRP) from the blood.

3. This PRP is then injected into specific areas of the vagina and clitoris. Virtually pain-free.

The potential benefits are impressive:

- Rejuvenation of vaginal atrophy
- Increased sexual desire and arousal
- Stronger and more frequent orgasms
- Increased natural lubrication
- Improved urinary continence
- Decreased pain during intercourse

The science behind The O-Shot® Procedure is based on the regenerative properties of PRP. The growth factors in PRP stimulate the production of new cells and blood vessels, rejuvenating the treated areas and leading to increased sensitivity and improved function.

PRP is used extensively in the orthopedic and oral surgery world as it is known for its healing and regenerative properties.

One of the great things about The O-Shot® Procedure is that it's a quick procedure with minimal downtime. Most women can return to their normal activities, including sexual activity, on the same day. And because it uses your blood, the risk of allergic reactions or side effects is very low.

I want to be clear: The O-Shot® Procedure isn't a magic bullet. Like any treatment, results can vary from person to person. Some women experience dramatic improvements, while others might see more subtle changes. It is essential to have realistic expectations and understand that it might take a few weeks to see the full effects.

The O-Shot® Procedurecan be particularly beneficial for women dealing with:

- Decreased libido
- Difficulty achieving orgasm
- Vaginal dryness
- Decreased sensation
- Painful intercourse
- Urinary incontinence

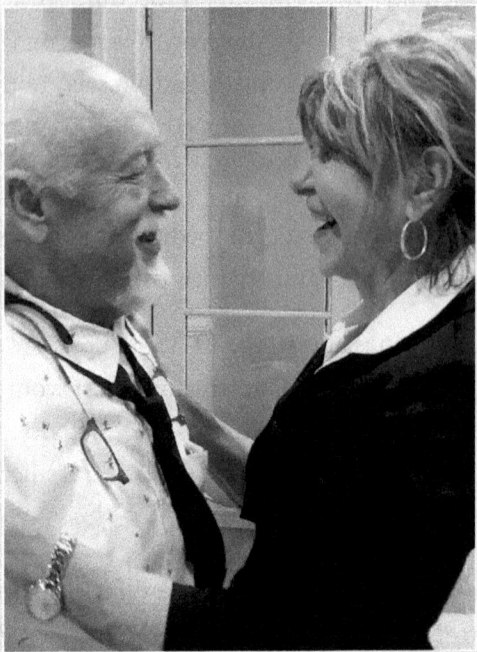

After getting The O-Shot® Procedure clitoral treatment, my orgasms are better, my vaginal dryness is gone, and I am no longer leaking urine. A true Win-Win Dr. Burkenstock!

~Angie W.

It's worth noting that The O-Shot® Procedure can be used in conjunction with other treatments. For example, I often recommend combining The O-Shot® Procedure with the HIFEM therapy, vaginal wand, and/or pelvic floor exercises, especially when dealing with incontinence issues.

I am frequently asked, "How long do the effects of the O-Shot last?" While experiences vary, many women report benefits lasting one to several years. Some clients choose to have the treatment repeated annually to maintain the effects.

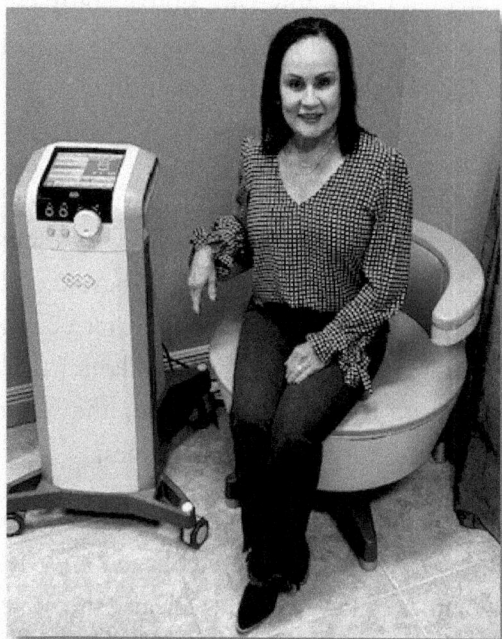

The HIFEM electromagnetic chair has significantly enhanced my quality of life. Working in a fast-paced environment requires me to be on my feet for up to 12 hours a day, and I previously struggled with frequent restroom breaks that disrupted my workflow. Since beginning treatment, I've experienced remarked improvement, my pelvic floor muscles are now stronger than ever, and those interruptions are no longer an issue. I am deeply grateful for Dr. Burkenstock and the HIFEM treatment for these life-changing results.

s~Countice L.

The HIFEM electromagnetic chair is a powerfully effective treatment for women of any age who have urinary leakage, orgasm issues, or vaginal atrophy and need to strengthen the pelvic floor. In a single 28-minute session, fully clothed and comfortably seated on the HIFEM chair, 11,000 powerful muscle contractions, Kegels, are delivered to the pelvic floor. Within six sessions, most clients report resolution of their urinary incontinence and enhanced sexual satisfaction.

These female scientific breakthroughs haven't gone unnoticed! Beloved Hollywood actress Drew Barrymore has always advocated embracing individuality and exploring innovative solutions. In recent years, she has become a vocal supporter of High Intensity Focused Electromagnetic Frequency Stimulation therapy. Oprah supports the ground-breaking innovation, the Vaginal therapy wand designed, to address pelvic health issues.

Red LED light therapy (600-662 nm) or near-infrared (810 nm) facial therapy is known to stimulate collagen and elastin to help your skin remain wrinkle-free and reverse the visible signs of facial skin aging. The result is smoother, healthier skin. A 2018 study shows that Red LED therapy is safe and effective against skin aging. This scientific breakthrough was transferred to vaginal rejuvenation too! When the red LED light is combined with heat and vibration, as in the Vaginal rejuvenation wand, it delivers renewing, age-reversing effects on the vagina and pelvic floor. Red LED light devices are a nonhormonal, noninvasive, pain-free approach to promoting pelvic floor muscle tone, sexual function, and intimate well-being.

Not all red LED devices are made equal, however. The specific wavelength of the red light (600-662 nm) plus the heat for improved blood flow and vibration are synergistic for sexual and vaginal health improvements. Red-light Vaginal devices are not overnight miracles; consistent use over time is key, so the more you use them, the better the result.

Sexual health is about more than just physical function. The O-Shot® Procedure can be a valuable tool, but it's most effective when used as part of a comprehensive approach to sexual wellness. This might include addressing underlying health issues, managing stress, maintaining open communication with your partner, and practicing self-care.

## YOU ARE SO WORTH IT!...

As we wrap up this chapter, I want to emphasize that you deserve to have a fulfilling and enjoyable sex life at any age. Whether it's The O-Shot® Procedure or another treatment option, don't hesitate to explore solutions if you're experiencing sexual health issues. Your quality of life matters, and more options are available now than ever before.

Sexual health is a vital part of overall health and well-being. A healthy sex life can improve your immune system, heart health, and self-esteem, and it can reduce depression and anxiety.

Keep reading to learn another cutting-edge approach to wellness: DNA testing for weight loss. This personalized approach to nutrition and fitness is revolutionizing how we think about weight management.

Ready to transform your life!
Scan or Call now to schedule a consult with Dr. Burkenstock

985-727-7676

# Chapter 9

## DARE TO BE THIN® DNA TESTING FOR WEIGHT LOSS: PERSONALIZED APPROACHES TO OPTIMAL WEIGHT

Welcome to the fascinating world of DNA nutrigenomics! Nutrigenomics studies how food and nutrients affect gene expression and health. This chapter will explore how your unique genetic makeup can influence your weight and how we can use this information to create personalized nutrition and fitness plans. This is cutting-edge information that is changing the game for long-term weight management.

Most traditional one-size-fits-all diets often fail. You've probably experienced this yourself when you try the latest fad diet that worked wonders for your friend, but you see little to no results. It's not because you're doing anything wrong; it's because your body is unique and responds to food and exercise in a personalized way.

This is where our simple DNA nutrigenomic testing comes in. By analyzing specific genes related to metabolism, nutrient processing, exercise response, and brain mutations, we can get valuable insights into how your body metabolizes food and burns fat.

## KEY AREAS IN WHICH DNA NUTRIGENOMIC TESTING CAN PROVIDE INFORMATION

- **Macronutrient metabolism**: How your body processes carbohydrates, fats, and proteins.

- **Micronutrient needs**: Your genetic predisposition for vitamin and mineral deficiencies.

- **Food sensitivities**: Genetic markers for gluten sensitivity, lactose intolerance, food allergies, etc.

- **Exercise response**: How your body responds to different types of physical activity depends on whether you are built with predominantly fast twitch, slow twitch, or equal proportions of each muscle gene type.

- **Eating behaviors**: Genetic influences include snacking tendencies, satiety, sugar cravings, and MTHFR mutations.

For example, in the DNA report, the glut2 mutation, if positive or turned on, means that one's sugar cravings are more than just a habit. This DNA type has an actual mutation for sugar cravings. We would use targeted supplements like our Sugar Smart, with berberine, and Omega Pure fish oil to support the urges produced by the glut2 mutation.

You might be wondering, "How does this help with weight loss?" Well, let me give you an illustration. Let's say your DNA test reveals that you have a genetic variation that makes it harder for your body to process carbohydrates. Armed with this knowledge, we might design a nutrition plan that follows the low carbohydrate percentage outlined in the DNA result and the higher percentages noted regarding healthy fats and proteins. A personalized approach is dramatically more effective than a generic, low-calorie diet.

Similarly, suppose your genetic profile shows that you respond better to high-intensity exercise for fat burning. In that case, we might focus your fitness plan on interval training rather than long, steady-state cardio sessions.

After years of dealing with excess weight, going to numerous doctors, and having a lack of self-confidence. I finally found Dr. Burkenstock. I joined her Dare To Be Thin™ weight loss program, and my life completely changed. I began my journey with Dr. Burkenstock in 2015, and I lost 82 pounds in my first year. My weight loss was accomplished without medications, and the "weight loss shots" were not yet developed. I am proud to say that in 2025, I am still 130 pounds. I have maintained a natural weight for my body type with her DNA-driven program and the custom supplements she provides. Thank you, Dr. Burkenstock

*~Xiomara*

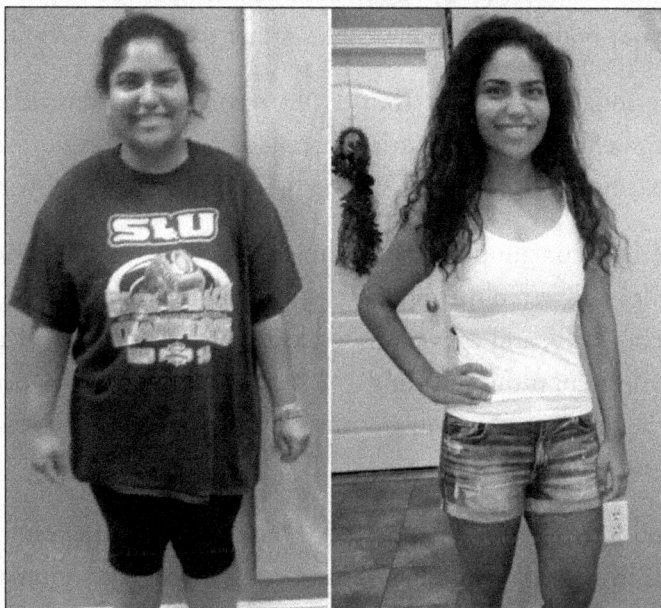

## DARE TO BE THIN® DNA NUTRIGENOMIC TESTING PROCESS

1. **Sample collection**: This is usually done with a simple cheek swab or saliva sample.

2. **Lab analysis**: Your sample is sent to a lab, where 28 specific SNP genes related to nutrition, fitness, and brain mutations are analyzed.

3. **Results interpretation**: A trained professional (like yours truly) reviews your genetic report.

4. **Personalized plan creation**: We create a tailored nutrition and fitness plan based on your genetic profile.

It's important to note that your genes are not your destiny; they are more like a blueprint. Having a genetic predisposition doesn't mean you're doomed to being overweight or that you can't enjoy certain foods. Instead, this information gives us a roadmap to work with your body's natural tendencies rather than against them.

My personal Dare To Be Thin® DNA testing report revealed that my most efficient macronutrient breakdown is a 1300-calorie daily intake consisting of 30% fat, 30% protein, and 40% carbohydrates.

My lifelong consumption of avoiding healthy fats—nuts and seeds, avocados, olives, olive oil, fatty fish (salmon, tuna, mackerel), dark chocolate, and eggs—was working against my DNA-derived macronutrient profile, making it very difficult to control my weight after beginning menopause—until I discovered this *invaluable DNA information.*

One of the most exciting aspects of DNA nutrigenomic testing for weight loss is that it can help us understand why past approaches haven't worked for you. For instance, if you've always struggled with low-carbohydrate diets, your genetic profile might reveal that you actually process carbohydrates efficiently and could benefit from a higher healthy complex carbohydrate intake.

An important note: Our bodies need all the macronutrients in some respect, and we should never have a no-fat or no-carb diet, etc.

## KEY BENEFITS OF USING DNA TESTING FOR WEIGHT LOSS

- **Personalized Nutrition**: Eat according to your genetic profile for optimal health and weight management.

- **Targeted supplementation**: Address potential nutrient deficiencies based on your genetic profile.

- **Best choice exercise**: Focus on the types of physical activity your body burns fat most efficiently with and responds to optimally.

- **Sustainable results**: Working with your body's natural genetic tendencies makes you more likely to see lasting results.

- **Improved overall health**: This approach isn't just about weight loss - it's about optimizing your overall wellness.

*A word of caution*: While DNA testing can provide valuable insights, it won't solve everything. It's a tool that we use in conjunction with a comprehensive plan with other essential factors like food allergies and sensitivities, blood sugar, thyroid hormone levels, and personal preferences to create a custom doable plan for each client. As with any health-related decision, work with a qualified healthcare physician who can help you interpret your results and create an appropriate plan.

## ─YOU ARE SO WORTH IT!... ──────

As we close this chapter, I want to emphasize how exciting this field is. We're moving away from generic, one-size-fits-all approaches to health and wellness and embracing personalized, science-based strategies. DNA genomic testing for weight loss is just one example of how we can use nouveau technology and scientific advancements to optimize our vitality and longevity.

Next, I'll share details about another treatment innovation that's making waves in the world of Anti-aging and aesthetics: Platelet-Rich Plasma (PRP) for non-surgical facelifts, hand rejuvenation, and hair restoration. Get ready to learn how we can use your body's own healing stem cells *To Turn Back the Hands of Time!*

Ready to transform your life!
Scan or Call now to schedule a consult with Dr. Burkenstock

985-727-7676

# Chapter 10

## PLATELET-RICH PLASMA (PRP) THERAPY FOR NON-SURGICAL FACELIFT, HAND REJUVENATION, AND HAIR RESTORATION

What if you could turn back the clock without going under the knife? Let's explore the world of Platelet-Rich Plasma (PRP) therapy and how it's revolutionizing facial, hand, and hair rejuvenation. This cutting-edge treatment harnesses your body's healing powers to restore youth.

First, a quick recap of what PRP is from our discussion of The O-Shot® Procedure. PRP is derived from your plasma. We draw a small amount of blood, process it in a special centrifuge to concentrate the platelets, and then use this platelet-rich plasma (PRP) for various treatments. Platelets are packed with growth factors and stem cells that stimulate healing and regeneration.

# PRP PROCEDURE

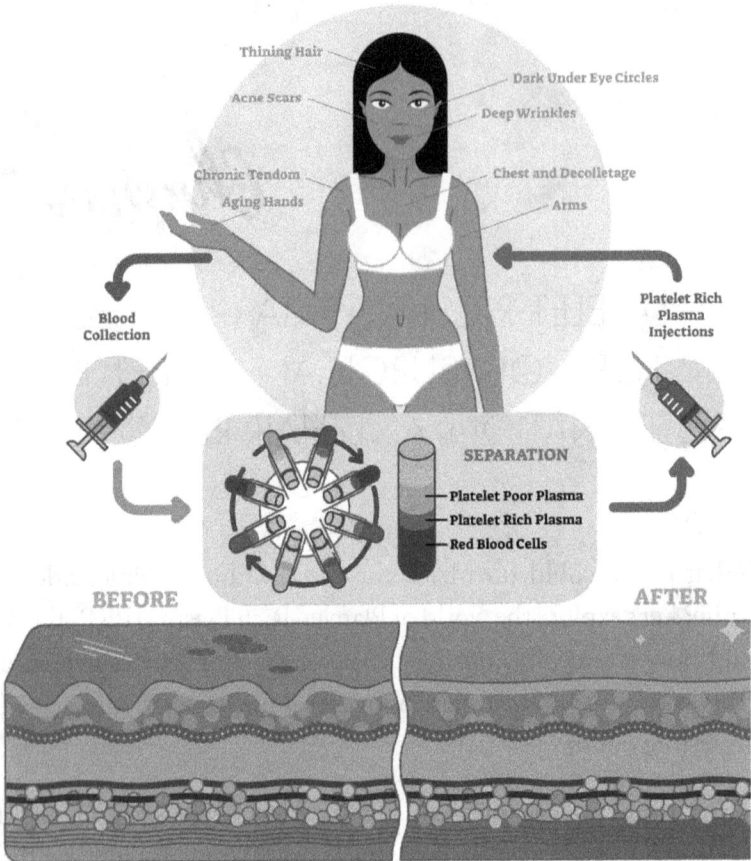

Thining Hair

Acne Scars

Chronic Tendom

Aging Hands

Dark Under Eye Circles

Deep Wrinkles

Chest and Decolletage

Arms

Blood Collection

Platelet Rich Plasma Injections

SEPARATION

Platelet Poor Plasma

Platelet Rich Plasma

Red Blood Cells

BEFORE

AFTER

Let's look at how we use PRP for facial rejuvenation:

## THE VAMPIRE OR PRP FACELIFT

Don't let the name scare you! This procedure combines PRP with dermal fillers like Restylane®, JUVÉDERM®, or Radiesse® to restore volume and improve skin texture and collagen fullness. Here is how it works:

1. We inject dermal fillers to sculpt and add volume for a more youthful face shape.

2. Then, we apply PRP topically and inject it into specific areas.

3. The PRP's stem cells and growth factors stimulate collagen production and improve skin quality.

## PRP VAMPIRE FACIAL

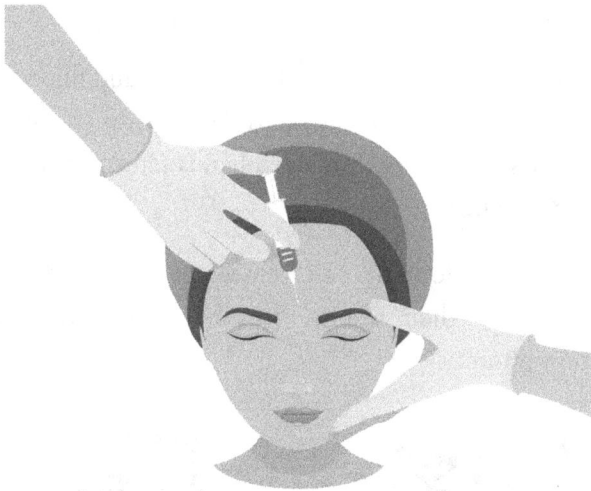

This is a less invasive option that involves microneedling with PRP.

1. Tiny needles create microscopic channels in your skin.

2. PRP is applied topically and injected under the skin, allowing it to penetrate deeply.

3. This stimulates collagen production and cell turnover.

4. PRP treatments are like adding seeds, fertilizer, water, and sunshine to a garden and watching the beautiful results unfold!

Benefits of PRP for facial rejuvenation include:

- Improved skin texture and tone

- Reduced fine lines and wrinkles

- Enhanced skin hydration and glow

- A natural improvement in appearance

### *Let's Applaud!*

Additionally, PRP is combined with light lasers and fillers to return volume and plumpness to aging hands. The treatment corrects age spots and hides veins. The thin, aged hands return to their former youthful appearance.

PRP hand rejuvenation offers an immediate result, and our clients are excited about their results. See the before-and-after hand rejuvenation photo.

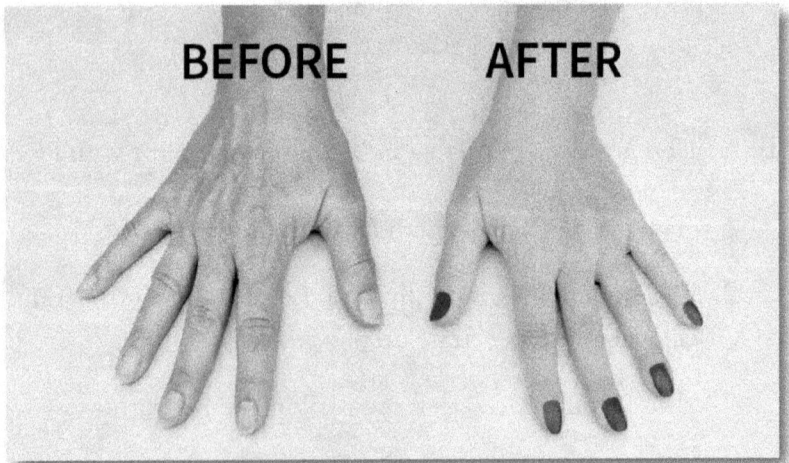

BEFORE    AFTER

# RESTORING A WOMAN'S MANE!

PLATELET-RICH PLASMA
(PRP)

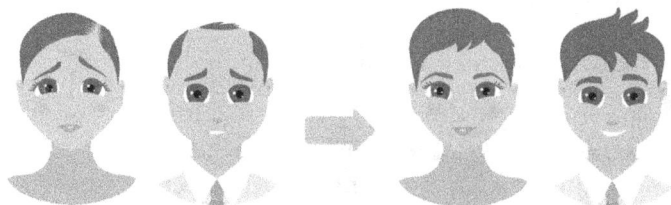

PROCEDURE

BLOOD COLLECTION

SEPARATION OF PLATELETS IN CENTRIFUGE

PRP INJECTION INTO THE AFFECTED AREA

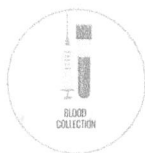

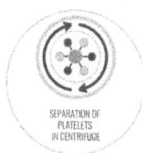

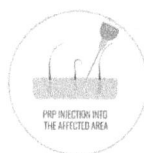

Also, PRP can help with hair restoration. Hair loss can be distressing for both women and men, and PRP offers a promising solution.

Here's how PRP works for hair restoration:

1. PRP is injected into specific circulation areas of the scalp.

2. The PRP's Growth factors and stem cells stimulate dormant hair follicles.

3. PRP can lead to increased hair thickness and new hair growth.

When injected into the scalp, the platelets in PRP become activated and release multiple growth factors, which promote hair growth.[1]

------

[1]Stevens J, Khetarpal S. Platelet-rich plasma for androgenetic alopecia: A review of the literature and proposed treatment protocol. International Journal of Women's Dermatology. 2018;5(1):46-51. doi:10.1016/j.ijwd.2018.08.004

PRP for hair restoration can be particularly effective for:

- Female pattern hair loss
- Male pattern baldness
- Thinning hair
- Alopecia areata (autoimmune condition causing hair loss)

One advantage of PRP treatments is that they are minimally invasive with little to zero downtime. Most people can return to their normal activities immediately after treatment. And because the treatment uses your blood, the risk of allergic reactions or side effects is negligible.

It's important to note that while PRP can produce impressive results, unlike hand restoration, it's not a one-and-done facial or hair restoration treatment. For the best results, we typically recommend a series of treatments spanning several weeks apart, followed by maintenance treatments as needed.

Here's a general timeline of what you might expect with PRP facial rejuvenation and hair restoration:

- **Immediately after treatment**: You might see mild redness or swelling, which usually subsides within a day or two.

- **2-3 weeks after treatment**: You may notice improvements in skin texture or hair *peach-fuzz* growth.

- **2-3 months after treatment**: This is when you'll typically see the full effects of the treatment.

While PRP is fascinating, it's not a panacea. It works best when combined with a comprehensive approach to skin and hair health, which might include:

- A professional skincare product line and good skincare routine

- Proper nutrition and supplements for healthy skin and hair

- Protection from sun damage with zinc and titanium sunscreen, as well as protective SPF clothing

- Stress management techniques

## YOU ARE SO WORTH IT!...

Aging is a natural process, and our goal is natural-looking improvements that help you feel more confident and vibrant so that you can be the most fabulous version of *YOU!*

As we close this chapter, I want to emphasize how thrilling it is that we can now harness our body's own healing power to address signs of aging. PRP represents a shift towards more natural, holistic approaches to aesthetic treatments.

Next up, another fascinating tool in our wellness arsenal: Heart Rate Variability Testing. This powerful diagnostic tool can provide valuable insights into your stress levels, homeostasis, and overall health. Stay tuned to learn how understanding your heart's rhythms can help you optimize your well-being!

DO MENOPAUSE MAGNIFICENTLY!

Ready to transform your life!
Scan or Call now to schedule a consult with Dr. Burkenstock

985-727-7676

# Chapter 11

## HOMEOSTASIS: HEART RATE VARIABILITY TESTING

### UNDERSTANDING STRESS AND HEALTH

Homeostasis is the state of Internal Balance, which is fundamental to the optimal functioning of the human body. It is measured by Heart Rate Variability (HRV). HRV testing is a powerful tool that can give us incredible insights into our homeostasis, overall health, and how our bodies handle stress. HRV is changing the game regarding understanding and managing our bodies' stress responses.

Contrary to what you might think, a healthy heart doesn't beat like a metronome with perfectly even spaces between beats. Instead, there's a natural variation in the time between heartbeats, which we call *Heart Rate Variability*.

Here's the key: Higher variability is generally a sign of better health. It indicates that your body is adaptable and resilient, able to respond quickly to changes in your environment or physical demands. Lower variability, on the other hand, can be a sign that your body is under stress and not adapting well. Low HRV indicates your body is living in the sympathetic domain—flight, fright, fight, or freeze—which prematurely ages the heart, brain, and other organs.

A high HRV indicates that your body is living on the parasympathetic side. Rest, repair, digest, and rejuvenate, extending life via homeostasis. **HOMEOSTASIS balance Is good health.**

So, how do we measure homeostatic imbalance and HRV? We use a specialized fingertip and toe sensor connected to a computer homeostasis program. The HRV report tells us your current homeostasis. If you are riding in sympathetic mode, we train the client's breathing and other techniques to accentuate the parasympathetic mode.

You might wonder, "Why should I care about my HRV?" Well, here are some of the incredible insights HRV wave testing can provide:

1. **Stress levels**: HRV is an excellent indicator of your body's physical and mental stress load.

2. **Recovery status**: It can tell us how well your body is recovering from exercise or other life stressors.

3. **Sleep quality**: HRV patterns during sleep can give us information about the restorative quality of your rest.

4. **Overall health**: Changes in HRV over time can indicate improvements or declines in your general health status.

5. **Risk of certain health conditions**: Low HRV has been associated with an increased risk of cardiovascular (heart) disease and cerebrovascular (brain) and other health issues.

One of the things I love about HRV Homeostasis testing is that it provides objective data about how your body is functioning. It's not just about how you feel; it's measurable, trackable information that we can use to guide your health journey.

One exciting area of HRV research is its potential use in predicting and preventing health issues. Some studies have shown that changes in HRV can precede the onset of certain health conditions, potentially allowing for earlier intervention.

## ─YOU ARE SO WORTH IT!...

As we wrap up this chapter, I want to emphasize that HRV testing is not about achieving a "perfect" score. Everyone's HRV is different, and what's most important is understanding your patterns and working to improve your body's resilience over time.

Our next chapter is near and dear to my heart: my own line: Skin Body Health Supplements designed to support skin, health, and natural hormone balance. I'll share the science behind these formulations and how they can support your life-long journey.

Ready to transform your life!
Scan or Call now to schedule a consult with Dr. Burkenstock

985-727-7676

# Chapter 12

## DR. BURKENSTOCK'S
## SKIN • BODY • HEALTH
## PRODUCT LINE

*\* Nourish Skin from Within*

*\* Natural Hormone Support*

*\* Improve Vitality*

*by Replenishing Your Deficiencies*
*Through Proper Supplementation*

We've discussed many exciting treatments and technologies, and now I want to share something very *personal* - my own line of medical-grade supplements designed to support your skin, vitality, and natural hormone balance from the inside out. I researched and developed my supplement line based on years of clinical experience in conjunction with biochemists and the latest science breakthroughs regarding anti-aging and women's health. Each vitamin in our product line is of the highest quality, is medical grade and carries the distinguished "GMP" seal of approval.

So, why are supplements so important, especially as we age? Even with the best diet, getting the proper nutrients our bodies need can be challenging. Plus, our bodies become less efficient at absorbing certain nutrients as we age. In addition, a leaky gut inhibits proper nutrient absorption. That's where custom-targeted supplementation comes in.

My Skin • Body • Health product line is designed to address some of the most common concerns I see in my practice:

1. Skin: preventing and treating photodamage

2. Hormone: Balance and support

3. Heart and Brain Health

4. Energy and Vitality: Enhancement

The following are some of the core supplements and why they're so beneficial:

## ANNATTO E

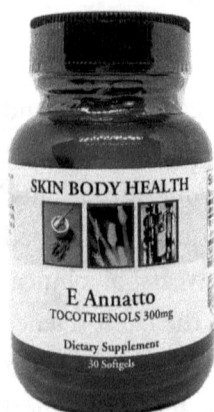

This powerful antioxidant is crucial for skin, liver, heart, bone, and metabolic health. This is not the tocopherol form of vitamin E; it is far superior. The tocotrienol-annatto form of Vitamin E protects your mitochondria and heart, fights cancer, and may improve diabetes, high cholesterol, enlarged prostate, and leaky gut syndrome. Annatto E reduces inflammation and oxidative stress from free radical damage, preventing premature aging. In my practice, I've seen remarkable improvements in skin texture when patients supplement with tocotrienol vitamin E.

## VITAMIN D

Often called the "sunshine vitamin," vitamin D is crucial for bone health, immune function, and even hormone balance. Proper vitamin D levels can help with mood, energy levels, and even vaginal health and male erectile function. Many adults report improvement in sexual desire and orgasm with Vitamin D support.

The prevalence rate of vitamin D deficiency is 40-80% of the population and is linked to several chronic diseases, including cardiovascular disease and cancer.

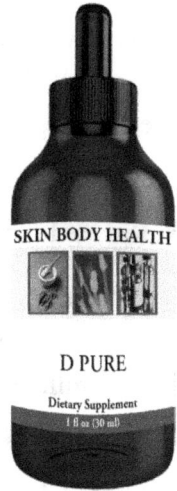

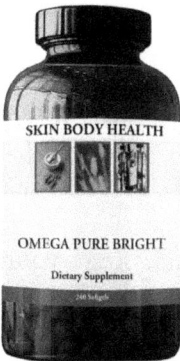

SKIN BODY HEALTH

D PURE

Dietary Supplement
1 fl oz (30 ml)

## OMEGA PURE FISH OIL

SKIN BODY HEALTH

OMEGA PURE BRIGHT

Dietary Supplement
240 Softgels

Rich in omega-3 fatty acids, it is a powerful anti-inflammatory that supports heart health, brain function, and, yes, even skin health. It can help keep your skin supple and may even help manage acne. High levels of the active ingredients, DHA and EPA, make this fish oil a powerhouse.

## DHEA

DHEA is the precursor hormone your body uses to produce other hormones, including estrogen and testosterone. As we age, our DHEA levels naturally decline. Supplementing with DHEA can help support overall hormone balance and may improve energy levels, mood, and libido.

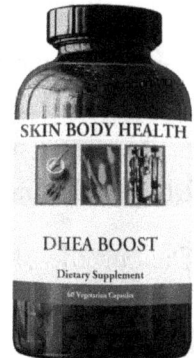

SKIN BODY HEALTH

DHEA BOOST

Dietary Supplement
60 Vegetarian Capsules

Let me emphasize that while these oral supplements can be incredibly beneficial, they work best as part of a comprehensive approach to health that includes a balanced diet, regular exercise, stress management, and proper sleep.

I typically recommend incorporating new supplements into your routine as follows:

- **Start with a baseline**: Before beginning any new supplement regimen, it's essential to get your vitamin, mineral, and hormone blood or urine levels checked to identify any deficiencies. This allows us to tailor the supplementation to your specific needs.

- **Start slowly**: Introduce new supplements one at a time. This allows you to monitor how your body responds and reveal any potential sensitivity.

- **Be consistent**: Supplements work best when taken regularly. It may take several weeks to months to see the full benefits.

- **Regular check-ins**: I recommend reassessing your bloodwork or urine and meeting with your Anti-aging physician every 3-6 months to ensure the supplements are working effectively and make any necessary adjustments.

Certain supplements should be taken at night for their best effect. For example, the liver makes cholesterol mainly at night, so cholesterol supplements should be taken after dinner, like Coq Ubiquinol, Omega Pure Fish Oil, and Annatto E.

One of the things I'm most proud of with my Skin Body Health line is the quality of the ingredients. We use only the highest-quality, bioavailable forms of nutrients and topicals to ensure optimal absorption and effectiveness. Of course, all our supplements are manufactured in an FDA-approved facility and carry the prestigious GMP seal of approval demonstrating they are safe, potent, and do their job. Our supplements undergo rigorous testing for purity and potency.

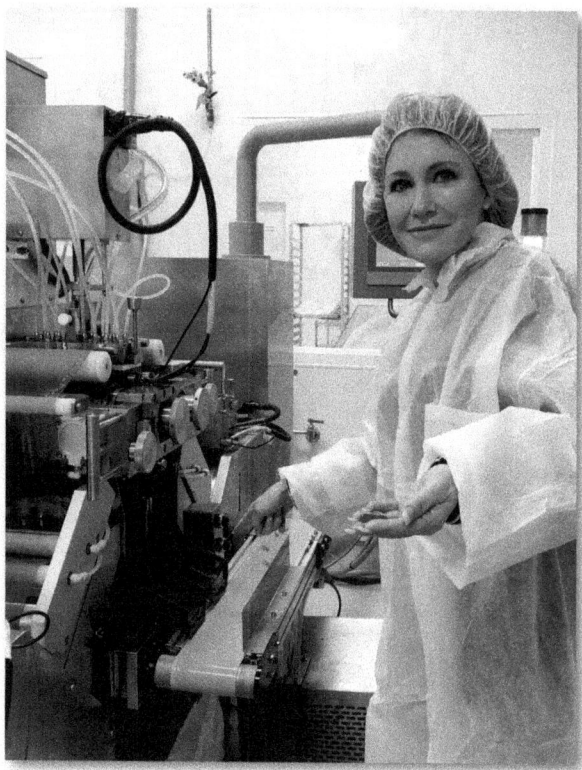

Dr. Burkenstock at her Skin • Body • Health manufacturing plant

There is much conflicting information about supplements, and figuring out what you need can be overwhelming. That's why I always recommend working with an Anti-aging physician who understands the complexities of vitamin deficiencies and hormone imbalances and can develop a personalized supplementation plan catered to your healthcare needs.

Ready to transform your life!
Scan or Call now to schedule a consult with Dr. Burkenstock

985-727-7676

# *Chapter 13*

## INTEGRATING WELLNESS AND BEAUTY

### THE PHILOSOPHY BEHIND DR. BURKENSTOCK'S PROTOCOL

Welcome to Part III of our journey! Now that we've explored the science of women's health and various treatments and therapies, it's time to tie it all together with my "Feel Fabulous—Look Fantastic" approach. This philosophy is at the heart of everything I do in my practice, and I'm excited to share it with you.

The core idea behind "Feel Fabulous—Look Fantastic" is simple: true beauty comes from within. When you feel magnificent, your body functions optimally, your hormones are balanced, and you're taking care of yourself, you will *Glow*. Conversely, looking your best can have a profound impact on your vitality.

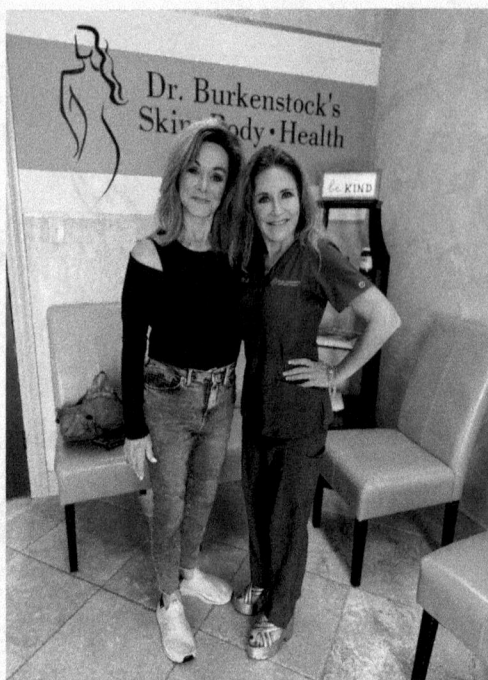

After giving birth to and raising seven children, I experienced years of weight and hormonal challenges. Under the care of Dr. Burkenstock , I have seen a remarkable transformation in my health and overall well-being. Her personalized weight management protocol and hormone therapy have helped me achieve and maintain a healthy weight of 125 lbs. at 5'4".

Through her guidance, I am now free of diabetes and high blood pressure, and my hormone levels remain well-balanced. Dr. Burkenstock's expertise, compassion, and commitment to women's health are unparalleled. She is a true leader in wellness and hormone replacement therapy, and I am deeply grateful for the care and encouragement she provides her patients.

~Kathy B.

The key components of The Burkenstock Protocol include:

- **Holistic Health (THE WHOLE YOU)**: I don't just focus on one aspect of health. Instead, I look at the entire picture: your physical health, mental well-being, sexual health, nutrition, sleep, stress levels, and more. Everything is an interconnected puzzle, and addressing all areas can dramatically improve your appearance and longevity.

- **Hormone Balance:** As discussed throughout this book, hormones are crucial to overall health and appearance. Balancing your hormones can improve everything from your energy levels, sexual wellness, and mood to your skin quality and weight management. Hormones also help you to say- Bye-bye belly Fat!

- **Targeted Treatments**: I use a combination of cutting-edge Western and Eastern treatments and time-tested therapies to address specific concerns. Whether it's PRP for skin rejuvenation, Bioidentical hormone therapy for menopause symptoms, or High-Frequency Electromagnetic Energy Stimulation for urinary incontinence and orgasm enhancement, we tailor the approach to your unique needs.

- **Nutrition and Supplementation**: What you consume dramatically impacts your appearance and energy level. We focus on nourishing your body from the inside out with a healthy diet and targeted supplementation.

- **Stress Management**: Chronic stress can wreak havoc on your health and appearance. Many studies show that stress is linked to many medical disorders, including Cancer. Did you know that even if you carry a particular cancer gene, it is only the *risk* of getting that cancer? *When the risk is* *combined with stress and high cortisol, then that cancer gene may turn on, and the disease presents itself.* We emphasize stress reduction techniques as key to vitality and longevity.

- **The Power of Positivity:** Taking time for yourself and cultivating a positive mindset is crucial for overall well-being. We help you develop self-care practices that fit into your lifestyle. Listen to positive motivation daily! Yoga, Pilates, hobbies, and time in nature all cultivate your inner spirit.

- **Feed the Senses:** Listen to music and Dance like nobody is watching!

Let's see how this works!

A middle-aged client presents to our clinic complaining of fatigue, weight gain, and dull skin. Instead of just suggesting a diet or prescribing a face cream, we take a comprehensive approach:

1. Start with thorough hormone testing to check for any imbalances.

2. Review daily food diary and bloodwork to recommend diet changes and specific supplements.

3. Evaluate HRV, cortisol levels, and daily stress and suggest stress-reduction techniques like meditation, yoga, and adrenal supplements containing Ashwagandha and Rhodiola, like our Adrenal Balance.

4. Possibly use treatments like The O-Shot® Procedure for vaginal rejuvenation or PRP facial revitalization, depending on the individual concerns.

5. Perform a thorough skin analysis and develop a custom skincare routine that treats any existing skin flaws.

By addressing the root cause of a client's concerns and taking a holistic approach, we can help her gain empowerment, which naturally translates to looking fantastic on the outside.

One of the things I love about this approach is that it's inspiring. It's not about chasing an unrealistic standard of beauty or trying to look like someone else. It's about being the best version of yourself – feeling vibrant, confident, and healthy at any age.

Here are some fundamental principles of the "Feel Fantastic - Look Fabulous" philosophy:

1. **Beauty is more than skin deep**: True beauty radiates from within when you're healthy and balanced.

2. **Age is just a number**: It's about how you feel, not the number of candles on your birthday cake.

3. **Small changes can make a big difference**: Consistent, small steps towards better health can lead to significant improvements over time.

4. **Self-care is not selfish**: Taking care of yourself allows you to show up better in all areas of your life.

5. **Everyone is unique**: What works for one person may not work for another. It's about finding the right combination for you.

Remember, *You Are So Worth It!* You deserve to feel vibrant, confident, and ravishing at every stage of life. My "Feel Fantastic - Look Fabulous" approach is about helping you unlock that potential and live your best life.

Next, we'll discuss Aging Gracefully, using mindset shifts and self-care practices that can help you thrive as you age. Get ready to redefine what it means to mature gracefully, like fine wine, which gets richer, more complex, and more valuable with age.

"Age is just a number.
It's totally irrelevant unless, of course,
you happen to be a bottle of wine."

— Joan Collins

# Chapter 14

## AGE GRACEFULLY: MINDSET AND SELF-CARE PRACTICES

In our youth-obsessed culture, it's easy to see aging as something to fight against. But I'm here to tell you that aging can be a beautiful, empowering process full of wisdom and spirit. We must flow with the tide, not against it, and approach it with the right mindset and self-care practices.

> Try to grab a hold of water, which will always elude you. It's soft, and yet it overcomes anything hard. Put the hardest substance —like titanium—and let water *flow* over it. Eventually, patiently and peacefully, the water will wear it away. Also, water will enter anywhere—through any opening at all. So, let yourself be like that.
>
> Like water, God is in nature, everywhere, and always. And we have so much to learn.
>
> ~Wayne Dyer

Aging is inevitable, and while we can't stop the clock, we can influence how we experience the aging process. It's about shifting our perspective and taking proactive steps to support our health and well-being. When Anti-Aging protocols are followed, we may be able to Turn Back the Hands of Time! Many Gerontologists have already won approval in the USA for the first-ever trial of a drug aimed at *treating aging* per se rather than any one of the individual diseases associated with aging. (A gerontologist is a professional who studies aging and promotes well-being among older adults, and their field of research is rapidly evolving into preventive medicine.)

Here are some primary mindset shifts to help you embrace aging:

1. **Focus on wisdom and experience**: You gain valuable life experiences and wisdom with each passing year. Celebrate that!

2. **Redefine beauty**: Beauty isn't about looking 20 forever. It's about radiating confidence, vitality, and elegance at any age.

3. **Practice gratitude**: Focus on what your body can do rather than perceived flaws or limitations. Welcome each day with "I get to..."

   I get to exercise...

   I get to read...

   I get to watch the sunset...

   I get to enjoy time with family and friends...

4. **Welcome change**: See aging as a new chapter in your life, full of opportunities for growth and new experiences.

**Start Today on the Burkenstock Protocol!**

Be 40 and Fabulous, 50 and Fantastic, 60 and Sexy, 70 and Sensational, and beyond! Let's grow young together!

Contact us at info@skinbodyhealth.com or skinbodyhealth.com

Many self-care practices can support healthy aging, such as:

- **Prioritize sleep:** Quality sleep is crucial for cellular repair, hormone balance, and overall health. Aim for 7-9 hours of sleep per night.

- **Stay hydrated:** Proper hydration is key for skin health, cognitive function, and overall vitality. Drink plenty of water throughout the day.

- **Move your body:** Regular exercise is a fountain of youth. It supports bone health, maintains muscle mass, boosts mood and memory, and helps manage weight. Find activities you enjoy and make them a regular part of your routine.

- **Nourish your body:** Eat a balanced diet rich in anti-oxidants, healthy fats, and lean proteins. Berries, leafy greens, fatty fish, and nuts support healthy aging.

- **Manage stress:** Chronic stress can accelerate aging — practice stress-reduction techniques like meditation, deep breathing, yoga, and even *intimacy*.

- **Stay socially connected:** Maintaining strong social connections is linked to better health outcomes and longevity. Make time for friends and loved ones.

- **Keep learning:** Challenge your brain with new skills or knowledge to maintain cognitive function. Take up a new hobby, learn a different language, or dive into a subject that interests you.

## LOW-DOSE NALTREXONE (LDN)

Anti-aging with Low-Dose Naltrexone (LDN) is a remarkable medication that has captivated the Anti-Aging community with its potential to restore vitality and promote overall well-being. We offer LDN as a transformative solution for clients seeking to optimize their health and slow down aging. Imagine a life where you can maintain youthful energy, enhance immune function, and reduce the risk of age-related diseases. LDN has emerged as a game-changer in the field of Anti-Aging, offering many benefits that can help you regain control over the aging process.

### BENEFITS OF LOW-DOSE NALTREXONE

- **Enhanced Immune Function:** LDN has been shown to boost the immune system, helping the body defend against infections, viruses, and other harmful invaders. By strengthening your immune response, LDN can help maintain your overall health and vitality.

- **Reduced Inflammation:** Chronic inflammation is a common feature of aging and a significant contributor to numerous age-related diseases. LDN has been found to reduce inflammation throughout the body, potentially alleviating symptoms associated with conditions such as arthritis, fibromyalgia, and autoimmune disorders.

- **Improved Mood and Mental Clarity:** Many individuals report experiencing improved mood, mental clarity, and overall cognitive function while using LDN. By stimulating the release of endorphins, LDN can positively impact mental well-being, promoting a sense of happiness and overall mental sharpness.

- **Alleviation of Chronic Pain**: LDN has been shown to provide relief for individuals suffering from chronic pain conditions, such as fibromyalgia, neuropathy, and migraines. By modulating pain pathways, LDN can help reduce pain levels and enhance your quality of life. LDN is usually prescribed as 1.5mg to 4 mg per day.

- **Improve Sleep**: LDN improves cortisol levels. Balanced cortisol levels improve sleep.

Another self-care practice: Loving your skin isn't vanity; it's sanity. Your skin changes as you age and needs different care than in your 20s or 30s.

## SKINCARE ROUTINE

1. **Cleanse gently**: Use a mild, non-drying cleanser to remove dirt and makeup without stripping your skin. We offer Rose Hip Seed Cleanser, made from rose petals and enhanced with olive oil Castille and vitamins A, C, E, and F.

2. **Exfoliate regularly**: This helps remove dead skin cells and promote cell turnover. But cleanse softly - over-exfoliating can irritate mature skin. Our Microdermabrasion Cleanser has silky, delicate crystals to enhance cell turnover gently.

3. **Hydrate, hydrate, hydrate**: Use a good serum moisturizer to keep your skin plump and hydrated. We offer Satin Seal for oily to normal skin, and our Squalane & Vitamin E serum for normal to dry skin. Don't forget to supplement with Omega Pure Fish Oil, Annatto E, and CoQ Ubiquinol to moisturize the skin from within.

4. **Protect from the sun**: Sun damage is one of the biggest culprits in premature aging. Use a broad-spectrum SPF every day, even when it's cloudy. Our Pure Mineral Sunscreen 30 SPF contains Titanium and Zinc to block the sun's radiation. It does not contain cancer-causing ingredients like benzene, oxybenzone, homosolate, and more.

5. **Night Repair**: Majestic Grape DNA Repair Serum, which repairs the skin's DNA telomeres with the power of Resveratrol from nature's grapes.

6. **Use targeted treatments**: Incorporate serums or treatments that address your specific skin concerns, whether fine lines, dark spots, or loss of firmness and elasticity.

**Dr. Burkenstock's personal favorites from her skincare line for mature skincare**

• Rosehip seed -cleanser

• Squalane & Vitamin E Serum- mosturizer for dry skin

• Microdermabrasion Cleanser- weekly exfoliator

• Majestic Grape DNA Repair Night Serum

Self-care rituals benefit your physical health, nurture your spirit, and help you feel centered. Some ideas include:

- Morning meditation or journaling

- Aromatherapy shower bursts (shower bath bombs)

- Regular massages or facials

- Nature walks or gardening

- Creative pursuits like painting, music, or dance

- Start comparing yourself to *yourself* (and no one else).

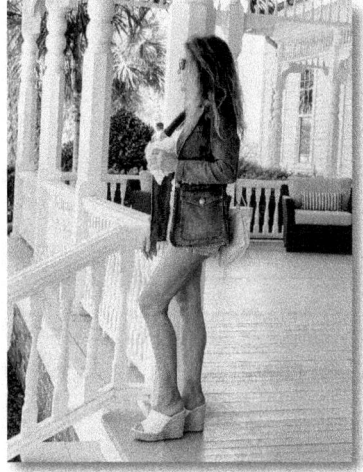

The key is to find practices that resonate with you and make them a regular part of your routine. These rituals can help reduce stress, boost mood, and contribute to an overall sense of well-being.

I love to walk every morning and give gratitude to God and the Universe. What a majestic world God has created for us.

To foster a more gracious mindset, remind yourself to say, "I get to" instead of "I have to."

For example, saying, "I get to wake up," "I get to take a walk," "I get to go to work," or "I get to take my loved one to..." helps you remember that these are opportunities you would miss if they were gone. It's a simple change that reminds you to be thankful and happy for things you usually take for granted.

As we wrap up this chapter, I want to emphasize that aging gracefully isn't about denying the reality of getting older. It's about approaching this natural process with positivity, self-love, and proactive care. It's about feeling comfortable in your own skin and radiating confidence at any age.

---

## There is a kind of beauty in imperfection.

### — Conrad Hall

---

**YOU ARE SO WORTH IT!...**

Aging is a privilege denied to many. Each wrinkle tells a story of laughter, and each grey hair a mark of wisdom gained. By shifting our mindset and prioritizing self-care, we can make these years the best of our lives.

In Chapter 15, I share beauty rituals and skincare regimens to help you maintain healthy, radiant skin as you age. I will also share the latest innovations in skincare technology and how to create a personal routine.

Ready to transform your life!
Scan or Call now to schedule a consult with Dr. Burkenstock

985-727-7676

# Chapter 15

## BEAUTY AND SKINCARE RITUALS FOR HEALTHY, RADIANT SKIN

Welcome back! Now that we've talked about embracing aging gracefully, we can dive into some practical ways to keep your skin looking radiant. Remember, healthy skin is beautiful skin, regardless of your age. It's not about looking 20 when you're 50; it's about having your healthiest, most luminescent skin possible at any age.

> I am 70, and I look great for my age. My decollete was the area that showed aging. I started Dr. Burkenstock's skincare line: Organic Pearl, Vitamin C, and Majestic Grape Serums.
>
> After she performed three sessions of the BBL/ IPL laser light treatments, my chest looks great. No more age spots or crepey skin.
>
> ~Cathy M.

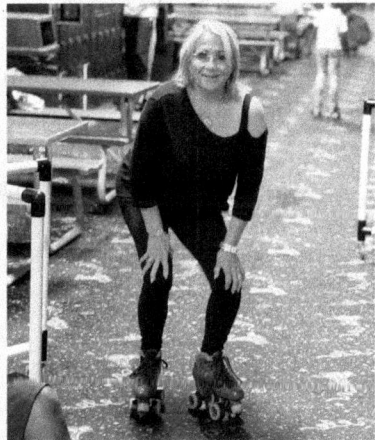

A comprehensive skincare routine consists of:

- **Cleansing**: Cleaning is the foundation of any good skincare routine. As we age, our skin becomes drier, so it's essential to use a gentle, non-stripping cleanser. Look for serums or creamy formulas with hydrating ingredients like rose hips, squalane, and Vitamin E.

- **Toning**: A good toner can remove any remnants of dirt or makeup, balance your skin's pH, and repair stress-damaged skin. Avoid harsh, alcohol-based toners that can dry out your skin. Instead, opt for hydrating, antioxidant-rich formulas that contain CoQ10, aloe, and chamomile extract.

- **Serums/Moisturizers**: Our skin produces fewer natural oils as we age, making a good serum moisturizer essential. This is where you can target specific skin concerns. Some key ingredients to look for:

  * Vitamin C, Wildberry extract, and kojic acid for brightening, pigment correction, and antioxidant protection

  * Squalane and Vitamin E for deep hydration

  * Hyaluronic acid and Coconut lipids for restoring critical moisture balance

  * Peptides for anti-aging, firming, smoothing, and DNA repair

  * Retin A /Retinol for cell turnover and collagen production

- **Sun Protection**: I can't stress this enough: SPF is your best defense against premature aging. Use a broad-spectrum mineral sunscreen SPF 30 or higher daily (rain or shine). The sunscreen should contain Zinc and/or titanium.

Wear a large-brimmed SPF protection hat and drape a scarf around your face to prevent sun damage.

## BEAUTY RITUALS THAT CAN TAKE YOUR SKINCARE GAME TO THE NEXT LEVEL

- **Weekly Exfoliation:** As cell turnover slows with age, regular exfoliation becomes more important. But be gentle! Over-exfoliating can damage your skin. I recommend a delicate crystal exfoliant like our Microdermabrasion Cleanser.

- **Face Masks:** A cleansing or firming mask can be an excellent weekly treatment for your skin. Look for clay-based masks with zinc, sulfur, collagen, and salicylic extracts. These masks draw out impurities that your daily cleanser may not reach deep within the skin.

- **Facial Massage**: This can help improve circulation, reduce puffiness, and promote lymphatic drainage. You can use your hands, a soft 2-inch (paint) brush, a jade roller, or a Gua Sha Stone.

- **LED Red Light Therapy:** This noninvasive treatment can help with everything from fine lines to acne. You can get professional treatments or invest in an at-home device.

- **Overnight Treatments:** Your skin does most of its repair work while you sleep. Take advantage of this by using rich night serums containing squalane and teprenone. These serums maintain the health of the skin's DNA telomeres, improving skin repair and cellular longevity.

# AND MY FAVORITE CORE FOUR!

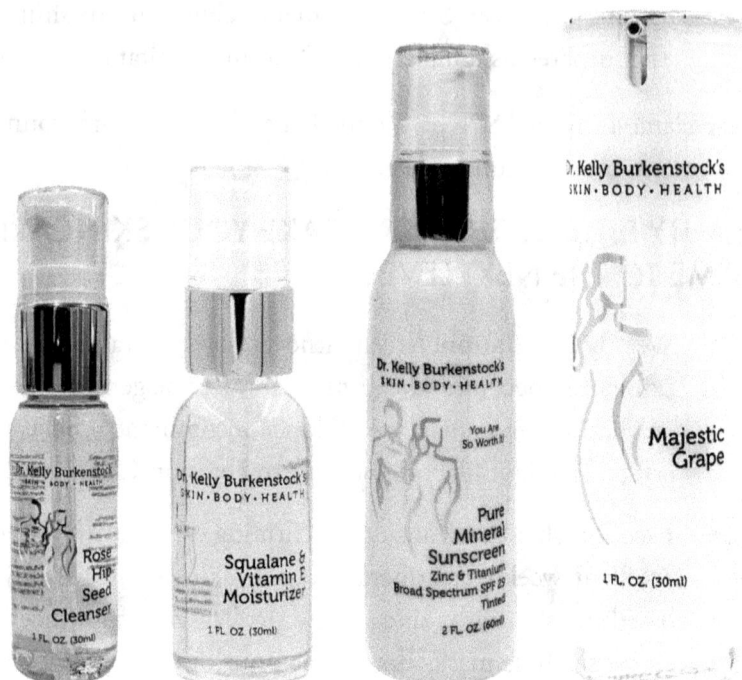

Dr. Kelly Burkenstock's
SKIN·BODY·HEALTH

Majestic
Grape

1 FL. OZ. (30ml)

Dr. Kelly Burkenstock's
SKIN·BODY·HEALTH

You Are
So Worth It!

Pure
Mineral
Sunscreen
Zinc & Titanium
Broad Spectrum SPF 25
Tinted

2 FL. OZ. (60ml)

Dr. Kelly Burkenstock's
SKIN·BODY·HEALTH

Squalane &
Vitamin E
Moisturizer

1 FL. OZ. (30ml)

Dr. Kelly Burkenstock's
SKIN·BODY·HEALTH

Rose
Hip
Seed
Cleanser

1 FL. OZ. (30ml)

**Dr. Burkenstock's Core Four Skin Care Favorites**

**Rose Hip Seed Cleanser:** A gentle cleanser enriched with a combination of Rose Hip Seed Oil, Olive Oil Castile, Seaweed, and Oil of Kumquat to nourish and protect the skin. It is rich in vitamins A, C, E, and F, which influence collagen growth and rejuvenation.

**Squalane & Vitamin E Serum Moisturizer:** This formula features squalane derived from olives, a pure and natural moisturizer. Olives and Vitamin E are among the most potent antioxidants and skin-protecting nutrients. Clear, see-through serums have fewer chemicals and preservatives and, thus, are better for reviving and reinvigorating beautiful skin. Cleopatra, known for her gorgeous skin, used serum from olives as a key component of her skin care regimen.

**Pure Mineral Sunscreen SPF 30**: a must-have! Using gentle yet powerful sunscreen daily is the key to anti-aging and protecting your skin. Our Pure Mineral Sunscreen is boosted with Zinc and Titanium to fight inflammation and protect your skin from the sun's UVA and UVB radiation. It is a true sunblock with a mild tint to prevent that white look. Only Titanium and Zinc guard your skin against photodamage, radiation, and Cancer.

A recent study in the medical journal JAMA showed that known cancer-causing chemical ingredients are found in many sunscreens. Oxybenzone and octinoxate were detected in the bloodstream after one single use. The study went on to prove that these toxic ingredients are also found in a woman's breast milk after using these sunscreens.

**Majestic Grape DNA Telomere Repair Serum:** This corrective serum targets multiple signs of aging and damaged skin to renew and rejuvenate while you sleep. It contains Resveratrol from red grapes, which protects the skin from oxidative damage. Majestic Grape visibly tightens and firms the look of aging skin while minimizing the appearance of discoloration and poor texture.

Medical-grade skincare products like ours at Dr. Burkenstock Skin•Body•Health are made with high-quality ingredients, containing more potent levels of beneficial ingredients like peptides and antioxidants that have been proven effective. Due to their superior potency, medical-grade skin care products are usually more cost-effective than over-the-counter products. They work best as part of a comprehensive approach to skincare that includes a balanced diet, hydration, regular exercise, stress management, and proper sleep.

Don't forget about the importance of what you put into your body. Your diet plays a massive role in your skin's health. Here are some skin-loving foods to incorporate into your diet:

- **Fatty fish**: rich in omega-3s for skin hydration and to reduce skin inflammation. Salmon, mackerel, and herring.

- **Avocados**: packed with healthy fats, vitamin E, and biotin to help achieve moisture and glowing skin

- **Nuts and seeds are rich in omega 3, vitamin E, and antioxidants**: Walnuts and almonds, for vitamin E and selenium, moisturize and reduce toxins. Sunflower seeds, flaxseeds, hemp, and chia seeds boost new collagen production.

- **Colorful fruits**: packed with anthocyanins, antioxidants, and Vitamin C, which help strengthen collagen fibers and reduce skin aging. Blueberries, raspberries, watermelon, and red grapes: (containing resveratrol) contain various skin protective antioxidants.

- **Colorful Vegetables:** Orange-tomatoes, sweet potatoes, and carrots contain lycopene and beta-carotene anti-oxidants that defend your skin from sun damage, signs of aging, and collagen breakdown. Green- spinach, kale, and broccoli contain vitamins A, C, and E, as well as iron and folate, which improve skin elasticity and youthful glow.

- **Green tea**: rich in catechins- antioxidants that boost blood flow to the skin and protect the skin from UV damage.

- **Dark chocolate (70% or more cocoa):** loaded with antioxidants that protect the skin from oxidative stress and flavanols that protect skin hydration and blood flow. Bonus: current studies demonstrate that dark chocolate decreases existing cholesterol plaque.

Hydration is also important. Aim for drinking at least eight glasses of water a day. You should invest in a good-quality water filter to prevent exposing skin to harmful contaminants.

This might seem overwhelming, especially if you're new to advanced skincare. Here's my advice: *start small*. Pick one or two new products or practices to incorporate into your routine. Give them time to work; it usually takes at least 4-6 weeks to see significant changes in your skin.

Remember, consistency is key. The best skincare routine is one that you'll stick with. And don't be afraid to adjust your routine as your skin's needs change. What worked for you in your 40s might not be as effective in your 50s or 60s.

> With Dr. Burkensock's tailored skincare program, Botox, and filler, I look at least 15 years younger. No one guesses my true age.
>
> *~K Spence*

As we wrap up this chapter, I want to remind you that while good skin care is essential, it's just a drop in the ocean. True beauty radiates from within. All the serums and creams in the world can't replace the richness of taking care of your overall health, managing stress, and cultivating joy in your life.

Coming up, we'll review lifestyle factors that contribute to optimal health and appearance.

## YOU ARE SO WORTH IT!...

Remember, your skin is your body's largest organ. Taking care of it isn't vanity - it's an integral part of your overall health. You deserve to feel confident in your skin at every age. Embrace these beauty rituals not just to look better but as a form of self-care and self-love. Because You Are So Worth It!

# Chapter 16

## LIFESTYLE CHOICES FOR OPTIMAL HEALTH AND BEAUTY

In addition to skincare and beauty rituals, lifestyle factors play a crucial role in how you look and feel. Remember, proper health and true beauty come from within, and your daily habits significantly impact your overall well-being.

### SLEEP

Let's start with the foundation of good health: sleep.

Sleep is not a luxury; it's a necessity. During sleep, your body repairs itself, balances hormones, and consolidates memories. Lack of sleep can lead to a host of issues, including weight gain and mood swings, and yes, it can even make you look older.

Here are some tips for better sleep:

- Stick to a sleep schedule, even on weekends.

- Create a relaxing bedtime routine. Dim lights an hour before repose. A hot shower or bath is helpful.

- Keep your bedroom cold, dark, and quiet.

- Limit screen time before bed. The blue light emitted by computers and cell phones can disrupt sleep patterns.

- Avoid caffeine after noon and avoid alcohol three hours before bedtime.

- There should be no reading in bed. We train our brains that the bed is for two things: Sleep and Intimacy!

I do not have a television or computer in my bedroom. The bedroom is for sleep and sex, much like a dog is trained to know when to eat or where to sleep. Our brain records patterns, and we must remind our brain what the bedroom is for.

## EXERCISE

Next, let's talk about exercise. Regular physical activity is crucial for maintaining a healthy weight, strong bones, good cardiovascular health, and a happy brain. But did you know it's also great for your skin? Exercise increases blood flow, which helps nourish skin cells and flush out toxins.

Aim for at least 30 minutes of moderate-intensity exercise five days per week. This could include:

- Brisk walking (Walk with weights for a belly fat burning, muscle toning crush!)
- Swimming
- Cycling
- Strength training (crucial for maintaining muscle mass as we age)
- Yoga or Pilates for flexibility and stress relief

Remember, the best exercise is the one you'll do consistently. Find activities you enjoy and make them a regular part of your routine.

## STRESS MANAGEMENT

Chronic stress can wreak havoc on your appearance. It can lead to inflammation, weight gain, hormonal imbalances, and even accelerate the aging process.

Some effective stress management techniques:

- Meditation or mindfulness practices

- Deep breathing exercises

- Regular exercise (yes, it helps with stress too!)

- Journaling

- Spending time in nature

- Engaging in hobbies or creative activities

- Planning events with family and friends

- Dr. Burkenstock's favorites are candles, music and dancing

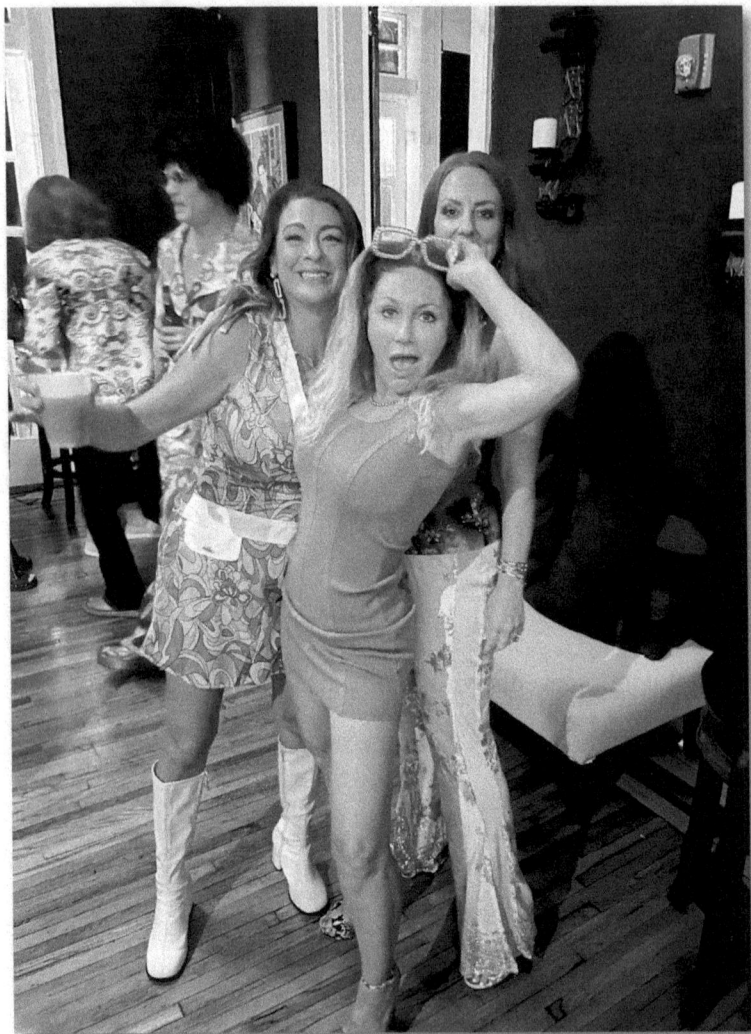

Deliah H., Jenae C. & Dr. B
Dancing for natural endorphins!

## NUTRITION

Of course, we can't forget about nutrition. What you eat doesn't just affect your waistline - it impacts your skin, hair, energy levels, and overall health. Focus on a balanced diet rich in:

- Lean proteins for collagen production.

- Healthy fats for skin hydration, hormone balance, and brain health.

- Colorful fruits and vegetables for antioxidants.

- Whole grains for sustained energy.

- Plenty of water for hydration.

Consider keeping a food diary for a week. You might be surprised at how your diet affects your energy levels and overall well-being.

## DR. B'S FOOD DIARY

### BREAKFAST: SWEET POTATO EGG BOWL

**Ingredients:**
1 sweet potato yam
1 cage-free brown egg
Fresh basil leaves
Paprika
**Directions**

Preheat oven to 425°F (220°C)
Poke holes in the potato skin with a fork
Line baking sheet with parchment paper
Place the potato on the sheet
Bake at 425°F for 45-50 min

Half the potato & scoop out the center
Place a raw egg in the potato bowl
Place in oven and bake at 425°F for 10-15 min
Remove and garnish with fresh basil & paprika
Enjoy!

Combining sweet potatoes and eggs creates a balanced meal, this keeps you full and balances energy levels throughout the morning.

## LUNCH: CHICKEN CAPRESE SALAD

**Ingredients:**

½ pound boneless, skinless organic chicken breast tenders
1½ tbsp avocado or virgin olive oil
1½ tbsp tamari, or Lea & Perrins Worcestershire (soy substitute)
1 tsp minced garlic
1 tsp Italian seasoning
¼ tsp black pepper
Fresh organic Spinach
Fresh organic Kale
Cherry tomatoes, halved
1 medium ripe avocado, sliced
Fresh mozzarella pearls- optional
Fresh Basil leaves (pressed/ mashed on plate for best flavor)

**Dressing**

Whisk together 3 tbsp Olive oil, 1 tbsp apple cider vinegar or balsamic vinegar, and 1-2 tsp of Dijon mustard. Add pepper to taste and set aside.

**Directions**

Preheat oven to 350°F (175 °C)

Mix avocado oil, tamari, garlic, Italian seasoning and black pepper in a bowl. Add the chicken and let it marinate for 10-15 min.

Bake chicken breast strips for 15- 20 min, on a parchment-lined baking sheet; flip halfway through.

Use a meat thermometer to ensure the thickest part of the strip reaches 165°F (74°C).

Remove the chicken strips from the oven and let them cool for 10 minutes. Don't cut until ready to serve, to keep them moist.

Wash, drain, and arrange spinach, kale, tomatoes, and avocado in a large bowl. Lay chicken strips and mozzarella on top. Garnish with basil leaves. Drizzle with dressing.

This salad offers a complete meal packed with proteins, vitamins and nutrients.

### DINNER: SALMON FILET & ASPARAGUS

4 (6oz) Salmon fillets
1 lb. asparagus stalks, ends trimmed
½ red and ½ yellow bell pepper sliced
2 tbsp extra virgin olive oil
2 lemons squeezed
½ yellow or purple onion, sliced into crescent rings
1 tbsp minced garlic
Black & white pepper to taste

## Directions

Preheat oven to 400°F (200°C)

Whisk together the olive oil, the juice of one lemon, garlic and pepper for the marinade and set aside.

Line a baking sheet with parchment paper

Arrange salmon fillets in the center of the sheet, skin side down.

Place asparagus spears, bell peppers, and onions around and atop the salmon.

Drizzle the marinade over the ingredients and place in the oven.

Place in oven and bake for 12-15 min, until salmon is opaque and flakes easily with a fork.

Asparagus should be tender-crisp.

Use a thermometer to ensure the thickest part of the strip reaches 135-140°F (58-60 °C)

*Optional*: Broil for the last 2-3 minutes to achieve a crispy, brown top.

To serve, squeeze the second lemon over the dish and garnish with fresh parsley or dill.

This dinner is full of Omega 3, antioxidants, and amazing Vitamins A, C, and K as well as B vitamins.

Bon Appétit!

## SOCIAL CONNECTION

Another lifestyle factor that often gets overlooked is **social connection**. Maintaining strong relationships and a sense of community is linked to better health outcomes and longevity. Make time for friends and loved ones, join clubs or groups that interest you, or consider volunteering at a nursing home, women's shelter, or pet adoption center.

## HABITS TO AVOID

In addition to positive lifestyle changes, there are also some habits to avoid:

- **Smoking**: It's terrible for your overall health and can accelerate skin aging.

- **Excessive alcohol consumption**: It can dehydrate your skin and disrupt sleep.

- **Prolonged sun exposure without protection**: This is a fast track to premature aging and increased skin cancer risk.

- **Crash diets**: can deprive your body of essential nutrients and lead to yo-yo weight fluctuations. This puts stress and strain on your organs.

Remember, it's all about balance. You don't have to be perfect all the time. The continuous everyday choices make the most significant difference in the long run.

Here's a challenge: pick one area of your lifestyle you want to improve. Maybe it's getting more sleep, adding a new form of exercise, or incorporating more vegetables into your diet.

> Lau Tzu eloquently taught, *"A journey of a thousand miles begins with a single step."*

Small, consistent changes can lead to big results over time.

As we wrap up this chapter, I want to emphasize that these lifestyle factors all work together. Good sleep helps you manage stress better. Regular exercise can improve your sleep quality. A balanced diet gives you energy for exercise. It's all interconnected.

As we continue exploring how to live your best life at any age, we'll discuss empowerment and self-advocacy in women's health. You deserve to feel confident and in control!

## ─YOU ARE SO WORTH IT!...

Remember, you are so worth investing in your vitality and longevity. These lifestyle factors aren't just about looking good; they're about feeling young, staying healthy, and living your best life at every age.

You've got this!

# Chapter 17

## EMPOWERMENT AND SELF-ADVOCACY IN WOMEN'S HEALTH

Welcome to Part IV! We've covered much ground, and now it's time to discuss how you can use this knowledge to advocate for yourself and live your best life. Because, let's face it, you are the expert on your own body and deserve to be an active participant in your healthcare decisions.

## SELF-ADVOCACY IN HEALTHCARE

It's about being informed, asking questions, and making decisions that align with your values and goals. It's about not settling for "that's just part of getting older" when you know something isn't right with your body.

## KEY STRATEGIES FOR BEING YOUR OWN HEALTH ADVOCATE

- **Educate Yourself**: Knowledge is power. Stay informed about women's health issues, especially those related to your age group and personal risk factors. My YouTube channel, Dr.BurkenstockSkinbodyhealth, and website skinbodyhealth.com, as well as Redefining Menopause. com, are valuable menopause resources with a vast array of mature female information. And remember, Dr. Google is not a substitute for professional medical advice!

- **Know Your Body**: Pay attention to changes in your body and track any issues. Consider keeping a health journal to note any patterns or concerns.

- **Prepare for Appointments**: Before seeing your healthcare provider, write down your questions and concerns. Bring a list! It helps keep your questions and thoughts organized.

- **Ask Questions**: If you don't understand something, ask for clarification. There's no such thing as a stupid question. Knowledge is power.

- **Seek Second Opinions**: If you're unsure about a diagnosis or treatment plan, it's okay to seek another opinion.

- **Understand Your Medications**: Know what you're taking, why you're taking it, and any potential side effects or interactions with other prescriptions or over-the-counter medication or supplements. Pharmacists have access to this information on their pharmacy software.

- **Bring Support**: If you're comfortable, bring a friend or family member to appointments to provide emotional support and help you remember important information.

**Tip**: Ask for a simpler explanation if the topic is too scientific or not understandable. Request a link or handout for further information.

## COMMON BARRIERS TO SELF-ADVOCACY AND HOW TO OVERCOME THEM

- **Fear:** Many women fear being seen as "difficult" or "high maintenance." Remember, a good healthcare provider wants you to ask questions and be involved in your care.

- **Time Constraints:** Healthcare visits can feel rushed. If you need more time, don't hesitate to ask for a longer appointment or a follow-up.

- **Lack of Confidence:** You might feel intimidated by medical jargon or doubt your comprehension. Remember, you are the expert on your body and you deserve the best.

- **Cultural or Language Barriers**: If English isn't your first language, ask for an interpreter. Many healthcare facilities provide this service. The new cellular phones have easy-to-use translation apps.

James and Lena G. were referred to me, they are both blind and have multiple medical conditions. They have been tossed around the medical system. Lena works as a grammar school teacher and does amazingly well. We looked at their layers of medications and discontinued many that were unneeded. We initiated vitamins and a safe exercise regimen for the couple. We taught them how to navigate and advocate for themselves. You do have a voice, and it deserves to be heard!

We should also address the importance of preventive care. Regular check-ups and screenings are crucial for maintaining health and catching any issues early. Here are some key screenings to keep in mind:

- **Mammograms**: yearly after age 40 to 75 or longer.

- **Pap Smears with HPV testing**: every 1 to 3 years after age 21.

- **Bone Density Scans**: every 2 years after age 65.

- **Colonoscopy**: every 10 years beginning after age 45. If a polyp or abnormality is found, more frequent testing is required.

- **Skin Cancer Screenings**: yearly beginning at age 35. Self-screening monthly at home is lifelong.

- **Blood Pressure Checks**: every 3 years, ages 18-39, and yearly after 40.

- **Cholesterol Checks**: every 5 years, ages 20-44, and every 1-2 years after age 45.

The specific recommendations for these screenings can vary based on age and risk factors, so discuss them with your healthcare provider.

Colonoscopies should begin at age 45 unless you have a first-degree relative with colon cancer, have been diagnosed with an inflammatory bowel disease, or have an inherited colon syndrome. Colorectal cancer screening can detect cancer before symptoms develop and has been shown to reduce death from cancer.

Mammograms should begin at age 40 and continue yearly. (Note: While some guidelines advocate stopping them at age 75, I personally recommend continuing them if a female is youthful and active and expects to live 10 years or longer. It is your body; you make the choice!)

Pap and HPV testing should begin at 21 and be repeated every 3 years. If HPV has been detected, more frequent Pap/HPV testing is recommended. HPV viruses are sexually transmitted and are the leading cause of cervical cancer.

*Key*: Bone density loss and osteoporosis risk factors include drinking alcohol, smoking, immobility (couch potatoes), being thin, lack of exercise, and medication side effects. Did you know that proton-pump inhibitor medications for acid reflux cause osteoperosis? Talk with your doctor regarding earlier Bone Mineral Density (BMD) screening if you have any of these lifestyle hazards.

Blood pressure is the silent killer; it often has no symptoms and goes undetected if not measured. High blood pressure increases your risk of heart attack, stroke, and kidney failure.

## BE EMPOWERED IN YOUR HEALTH JOURNEY

- **Trust your instincts**: Speak up if something doesn't feel right.

- **Make informed decisions**: Weigh the pros and cons of different treatment options.

- **Take an active role in your health**: Implement lifestyle choices, not just medical treatments.

- **Set boundaries**: It's okay to say no to treatments you're uncomfortable with. Consult with more than one physician and more than one *Type* of physician- Western and Eastern medicine. For example, Anti-Aging, Functional, or Integrative medicine in addition to primary care or adult Internal medicine.

- **Celebrate your body**: Focus on what your body can do, improve flexibility with yoga, Pilates, and Tai Chi, and practice mindfulness and meditation.

Remember, empowerment isn't about doing everything on your own. It's about being an active partner in your healthcare team.

Anti-aging medicine is a medical science that aims to treat the underlying causes of aging and extend the healthy lifespan of humans. Anti-aging physicians use a holistic and integrative approach to treating body and mind via lifestyle modification, fitness coaching, nutrition and exercise protocols, acupuncture, osteopathic, and massage therapy. This methodology empowers clients to look phenomenal and feel vivacious at any age!

## YOU ARE SO WORTH IT!...

As we wrap up this chapter, I emphasize that you can develop self-advocacy and fortitude skills over time. Start small if you need to. Maybe it's asking one question at your next appointment or researching a health topic that interests you. Every step you take towards being more involved in your healthcare is a step towards living your empowered life.

In the following chapter, we'll discuss how to create a personalized wellness plan incorporating all the elements we've discussed. We'll discuss setting realistic goals, creating sustainable habits, and adjusting your plan as your personal needs change.

> "I learned a long time ago the wisest thing I can do is be on my own side, be an advocate for myself and others like me."
>
> ~Maya Angelou

Ready to transform your life!
Scan or Call now to schedule a consult with Dr. Burkenstock

985-727-7676

# Chapter 18

## CREATING YOUR PERSONALIZED WELLNESS PLAN

We've covered a lot of ground, and it's time to pull it all together to create a personalized wellness plan that works distinctively for *you*. Remember, there's no one-size-fits-all approach to health, beauty, and wellness. What works for your best friend or sister might not fit you best. Designing a plan tailored to your unique needs, goals, and lifestyle is essential.

The following maps out the process of creating your personalized wellness plan:

## 1. PRIORITIZE YOUR FOCUS AREAS

This might include:

- Hormone balance
- Stress management
- Nutrition
- Exercise
- Sleep Quality

- Skin Rejuvenation
- Weight loss
- Sexual satisfaction
- Improving relationships

## 2. SET CLEAR, REALISTIC GOALS

Be specific and realistic. Instead of "I want to be healthier," try something like:

- "I want to walk/ bike 20 minutes per day."
- "I want enough energy to walk up a flight of stairs or play with my grandkids without getting winded."
- "I want to reduce my hot flashes by 50%."
- "I want to lose 5 pounds in a month."

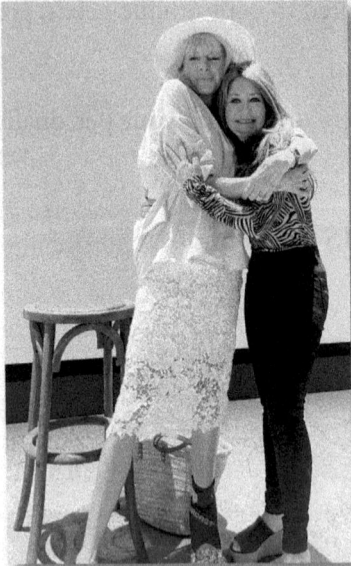

Ibiza, Spain

# Remember, your mind does what it thinks you want it to do.

~Marisa Peer,
Author, "I Am Enough"

## 3. CREATE ACTION STEPS

For each focus area, create specific, actionable steps.

- **Hormone balance**: Schedule hormone bloodwork and consult your Anti-aging hormone physician.

- **Stress management**: Start a daily 10-minute meditation practice. There are many free ones online or on YouTube.

  {I recommend "A Meditation for Self-Love: Free Guided Meditation" by Headspace and "Meditate: Be Present" by Daily Calm.}

- **Nutrition**:

  - Add one serving of vegetables or salad to each meal.

  - Add one glass of water before each meal.

  - Put your fork down between bites.

  - Use a small plate.

These steps will allow you to feel full faster and eat less.

## 4. BUILD IN ACCOUNTABILITY

How will you stay on track?

- Keep a simple journal or use a health-tracking app.

- Finding a wellness buddy or group.

- Schedule regular check-ins with your Anti-Aging physician.

## RECOMMENDED HEALTHCARE TRACKING APPS

- **YUKA (free)**: instantly scans barcodes of food and cosmetic products to assist you in making healthier food and personal care product choices.

- **Headspace (free)**: offers meditation exercises and health-tracking features.

## 5. PLAN FOR OBSTACLES

Think about potential challenges and how you'll handle them. If you know you struggle with emotional eating when stressed, what healthy coping mechanisms can you implement? For example, a five-minute walk around the office or neighborhood or 20 jumping jacks will release happy brain endorphins and, often, cut the cravings for comfort food.

## 6. INCLUDE SELF-CARE AND JOY

Your wellness plan should feel like self-love – a gift to yourself. Include activities that bring you bliss and help you relax. This might be a 20-minute daily music or dance ritual, a monthly massage, or creating space for a hobby you love.

## 7. MAKE IT SUSTAINABLE

The best wellness plan is one you can maintain. Consistency is key. Start small and gradually build up. It's better to make one small change that sticks than to overhaul your entire life and burn out in a week.

**You will face many defeats in life,**
**But never let yourself be defeated!**

~Maya Angelou

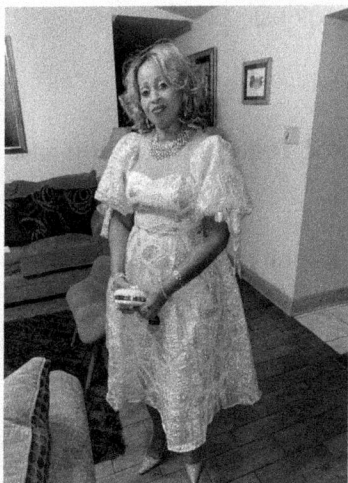

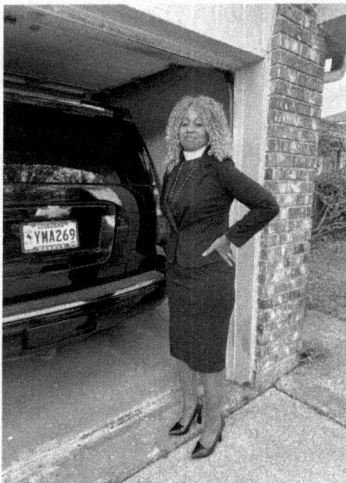

I lost over a hundred pounds with the support of Dr. B. I changed my diet, got up every morning, and walked 4 miles before work for the last 10 years. I feel superb, I look great, and I am living my best life.

*~Evelyn S.*

1.  **Be Flexible**: Revising your plan is okay if something isn't working. Your needs may change over time, and your lifestyle plan should evolve with you.

2.  **Celebrate Small Wins**: Acknowledge and celebrate your progress, no matter how small it might seem. Give yourself a "High 5" in the mirror every morning.

## Top Motivational Tips to Remember

Motivation is internal. If you believe you will succeed or fail, you're right!

Hang out with Superstars; it's contagious!

Proceed as if Success is Inevitable ~Blake Johnson

Challenge yourself with a DAILY goal. **Today**, I will do this ONE thing to make **today** a success!

Motion creates emotion. ~Tony Robbins. Get up and make things happen!

Creating a wellness plan is not about achieving perfection. It's about making conscious choices that support your health and well-being.

## YOU ARE SO WORTH IT!...

As we wrap up this chapter, I want to emphasize that your wellness journey is uniquely yours. Don't compare yourself to others or get caught up in what you "should" be doing. Focus on what makes you feel good, what aligns with your values, and what helps you live your best life.

Our next chapter will discuss navigating aging with confidence and vitality.

# Chapter 19

## NAVIGATING AGING WITH CONFIDENCE AND VITALITY

Here's the truth: getting older is inevitable, but how you experience aging is primarily up to you. It's time to rewrite the narrative around aging and embrace this stage of life with open arms.

Society is obsessed with youth. We're bombarded with messages that tell us aging is something to fear or fight against. But I'm here to tell you that aging can be a beautiful and empowering process if approached with the right attitude.

---

### "Youth Is the gift of nature, but age is a work of art."

~Stanislaw Jerzy Lec

---

## KEY MINDSET SHIFTS TO HELP YOU NAVIGATE AGING WITH CONFIDENCE

1. **Embrace Your Wisdom**: With age comes experience and knowledge. Celebrate the wisdom you've gained over the years.

2. **Focus on Possibilities, Not Limitations**: Instead of thinking about what you can't do, focus on all the things you can do and the new opportunities that come with this stage of life.

3. **Practice Self-Compassion**: Be kind to yourself. Your body is changing, and that's okay. Treat yourself with the same compassion you'd offer a dear friend.

4. **Redefine Beauty**: Beauty isn't about looking 30 forever. It's about radiating confidence, joy, and vitality at any age.

5. **Cultivate Gratitude**: Focus on what you're grateful for. This can shift your perspective and increase overall life satisfaction.

I have learned that being adaptable and optimistic reduces stress and allows for a longer and happier life. Research has also shown that it pays to be a little stubborn! *Stubborn people actually live longer.*

## MAINTAINING VITALITY AS YOU AGE

1. **Stay Physically Active**: Regular exercise is crucial for maintaining strength, flexibility, and overall health. Find activities you enjoy and make them a regular part of your routine.

2. **Keep Your Mind Sharp**: Engage in activities that challenge your brain. This could be learning a new language or skill, doing puzzles, or taking up a new hobby.

3. **Maintain Social Connections**: Strong social ties are linked to better health outcomes and longevity. Make time for friends and family, and don't hesitate to form new connections.

4. **Eat a Nutrient-Dense Diet**: Our nutritional needs change as we age. Focus on 'whole' foods that provide the nutrients your body needs to thrive. Colored foods are healthiest as they contain vitamins, minerals, antioxidants, and fiber. Remember that fresh is best! Don't overcook or laden vegetables with heavy sauces and oils.

5. **Prioritize Sleep**: Good sleep is crucial for overall health and cognitive function. Aim for 7-9 hours of quality sleep each night. Keep your bedroom dark, cold, and quiet—no TV, computers, or reading in bed. The bedroom should be used for only two activities: sleep and intimacy.

6. **Manage Stress**: Chronic stress can accelerate aging. Practice stress-reduction techniques like meditation, yoga, or deep breathing exercises.

## SOCIAL CONNECTIONS IN AGING

We all know that a balanced diet and exercise are essential for staying healthy. However, a growing body of research shows that social connections are another factor that is even more critical for keeping us in good physical and mental shape.

A landmark study published in 2010 found that the quality of someone's relationships is a more significant predictor of early death than obesity and physical inactivity and on par with smoking and alcohol consumption.[1]

"The size of these effects really can't be overstated; they're enormous," says Tegan Cruwys, an associate professor and clinical psychologist at the Australian National University.

A sense of purpose can positively contribute to well-being and life satisfaction as we age. This could involve:

- Volunteering for a cause you care about

- Mentoring younger individuals in your field

- Pursuing a long-held dream or project you are passionate about

- Spending time with family and friends and handing down family traditions

Remember, it's never too late to try something new or pursue a life-long goal. Age should not be a barrier to living a fulfilling life.

---

[1] https://www.ncbi.nlm.nih.gov/pmc/articles/PMC2910600

## IT IS NEVER TOO LATE!

Louise Hay was an inspirational teacher and self-help pioneer who wrote and published the bestseller *You Can Heal Your Life.*

At age 62, Louise began a small venture in her living room, eventually becoming Hay House, Inc., the world's largest publisher of self-help books, events, and courses.

## COMMON CONCERNS ABOUT AGING AND HOW TO HANDLE THEM

- **Health Concerns**: Stay proactive about your health. Regular check-ups and screenings are crucial. Don't hesitate to discuss any concerns with your healthcare provider.

- **Changes in Appearance**: Focus on overall health and well-being rather than trying to look twenty. To celebrate your changing appearance, you can do some beauty enhancements with micro-dermabrasion, laser, or Botox if you choose. But remember, you are fabulous just the way you are!

- **Loss of Independence**: Stay active and engaged to maintain your independence as long as possible. If you need help, remember that accepting support is a sign of strength, not weakness.

- **Financial Concerns**: It's never too late to improve your financial literacy. Consider consulting with a banker or financial advisor to help you plan.

- **Loneliness**: Combat loneliness by staying socially active. Consider joining clubs, taking classes, or volunteering to meet like-minded individuals.

## Dr. Burkenstock's approach to aging

Find that balance between accepting we are getting older without succumbing to cultural definitions of who we should be at age 50, 60, 70, and beyond.

As we wrap up this chapter, I want to emphasize that aging with confidence and vitality is more than just physical health. It's about nurturing all aspects of one's well-being—mental, emotional, and spiritual.

Remember, you have the power to shape your aging experience. You can make these years the best of your life by maintaining a positive mindset, staying active and engaged, and caring for your overall health.

In the final chapter, I'll share some inspiring testimonials and success stories from women who have transformed their lives using the Burkenstock Protocol. These stories will show you that it's never too late to take control of your health and live your most magnificent life.

**Thoughts on aging and beauty, Dr. Burkenstock and Karen S.**

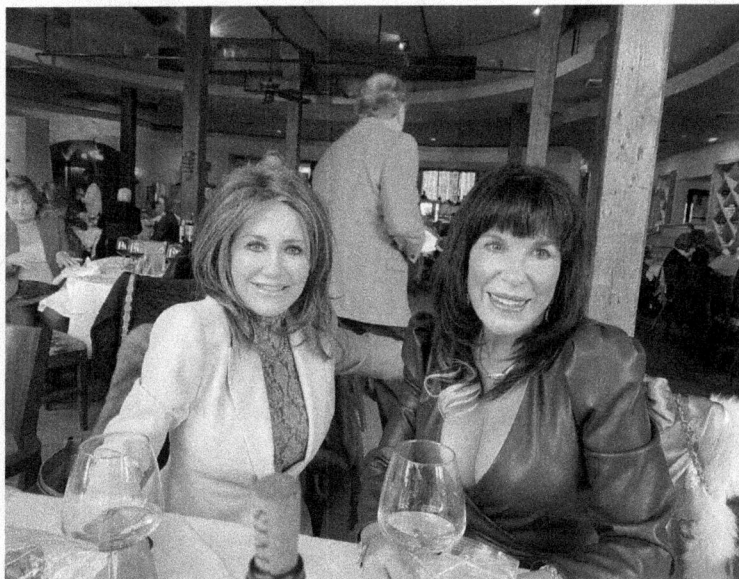

I began going to Dr. Burkenstock at 65; I was menopausal, lacked confidence, and just felt old. Dr. Burkenstock ordered bloodwork, and the results showed I had zero hormones, even though I was on the estrogen hormone patch. I began her bioidentical hormones, the true cascade, and my mind felt better and happier. I got the spring back in my step. I added her Skincare regimen, and the glow returned to my face.

I feel terrific and look phenomenal.

~Karen S.

## YOU ARE SO WORTH IT!...

Your age is not a limitation; it's a testament to your resilience, wisdom, and the rich life you've lived. Let's continue to grow, learn, and thrive together!

~Dr. Burkenstock

Ready to transform your life!
Scan or Call now to schedule a consult with Dr. Burkenstock.

985-727-7676

# Chapter 20

## TESTIMONIALS AND SUCCESS STORIES: REAL-LIFE TRANSFORMATIONS WITH DR. BURKENSTOCK'S PROTOCOL

Welcome to our final chapter! We've explored various aspects of women's health, wellness, and aging. I will share some inspiring stories from real women who have transformed their lives using Dr. Burkenstock's Protocol. These stories testify to the power of taking control of your health and incorporating a holistic approach to wellness.

### STORY 1: SARAH'S HORMONE BALANCE JOURNEY

Sarah, 52, came to me struggling with severe menopausal symptoms. Her hot flashes, mood swings, and insomnia were negatively impacting her quality of life.

"I felt like I was losing myself," Sarah shared. "I couldn't sleep, I was always irritable, and I just didn't feel like me anymore."

We started Sarah on a personalized bioidentical natural hormone replacement therapy plan, combined with lifestyle changes, including her Dare to Be Thin™ DNA-driven diet and regular yoga practice. We also incorporated customized medical-grade supplements to support her overall health.

Within three months, Sarah reported a dramatic improvement in her symptoms. "I feel like I've got my life back," she said. "My hot flashes are gone. I'm sleeping through the night and have energy again. Dr. Burkenstock's Protocol didn't just treat my symptoms; it helped me feel like myself again."

Sarah's plan began with comprehensive bloodwork, including an extensive hormone profile. This allowed me to evaluate her blood sugar, thyroid, cholesterol, inflammation, and major organ status. I discovered her personal vitamin and mineral deficiencies and developed a custom hormone treatment plan to rebalance her hormone cascade.

## STORY 2: LISA'S WEIGHT LOSS SUCCESS

Lisa, 48, had been struggling with weight gain and fatigue for years. She couldn't shift the extra pounds despite trying various diets and exercise programs.

We started by doing comprehensive hormone testing and discovered that Lisa had an underactive, slow thyroid and insulin resistance. We developed a personalized plan that included thyroid support and dietary changes to balance her blood sugar (avoiding white foods, such as bread, rice, pasta, potatoes, and sugar) and incorporated a tailored exercise program. Her Dare to Be Thin™ DNA report recommended specific exercise regimens for her to burn fat more efficiently.

"Dr. Burkenstock's Protocol was so different from anything I'd tried before," Lisa said. "For the first time, I felt like someone was looking at me as a whole person, not just a number on a scale."

Over six months, Lisa lost 30 pounds, was down two dress sizes, and saw improvements in her energy levels. More importantly, she felt empowered to take control of her health.

"I'm not just thinner; I'm healthier and happier," Lisa shared. "I've learned so much about my body and how to care for myself. This isn't just a diet; it's a whole new way of living."

Lisa followed the seven steps to Skinny Success Weight Loss Wheel® by Dr. Burkenstock.

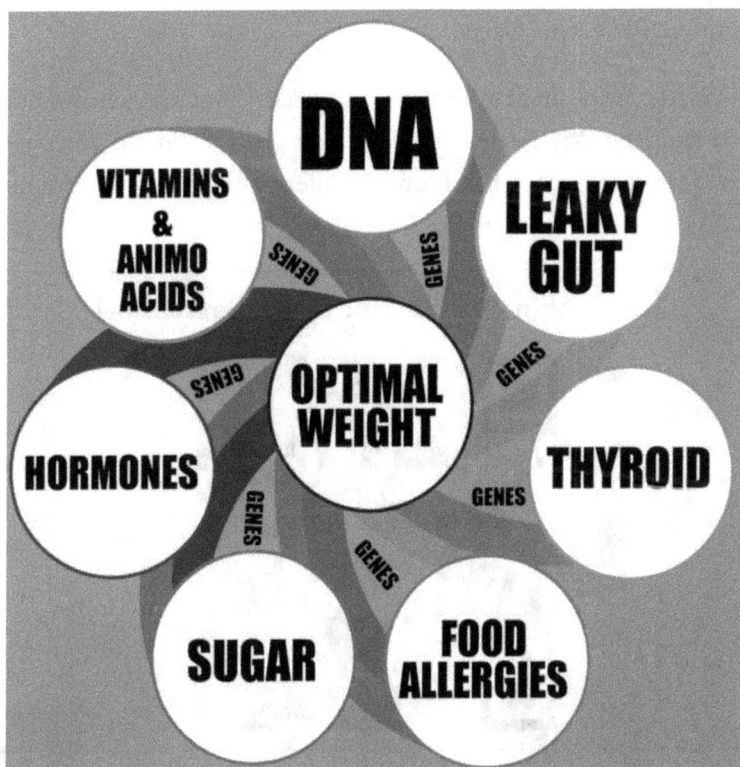

## STORY 3: MARIA'S SKIN TRANSFORMATION

Maria, 60, came to me concerned about the changes she saw in her skin. She felt like she had aged dramatically in just a few years and was losing confidence.

We approached Maria's concerns from multiple angles and started her on a customized skincare routine, including targeted treatments for her specific concerns. We reviewed her nutrition, recommending foods rich in antioxidants and healthy fats to support skin health from the inside out.

We also incorporated innovative treatments like PRP (platelet-rich plasma) facials and BBL/IPL (Broad Band Light) laser to stimulate collagen production. Later, we added a little Botox and Filler to complete the masterpiece.

"I was skeptical at first," Maria admitted. "But the results have been amazing. My face looks better now than it did ten years ago. But more than that, I feel more confident and comfortable in my own skin."

**Maria's Skin Care Routine by Dr. Burkenstock**

| AM: | Dr. Burkenstock's Rose Hip Seed Cleanser, Satin Seal Moisturizer, and Pure Mineral Sunscreen |
|---|---|
| PM: | Dr. Burkenstock's Rose Hip Seed Cleanser, COQ Toner, and Retin A mixed with Majestic Grape DNA Repair Serum |
| Weekly: | Dr. Burkenstock's Microdermabrasion Cleanser followed by her Beta Salicylic Exfoliator |

## STORY 4: JENNIFER'S JOURNEY TO VITALITY

Jennifer, 72, came to me feeling generally unwell. She had low energy, was having trouble sleeping, and felt like she had "brain fog" most of the time.

After comprehensive testing, we discovered that Jennifer had several nutrient deficiencies and hormonal imbalances. We created a personalized supplement plan to address her deficiencies, began bio identical hormone creams, and implemented lifestyle changes to support her overall health.

"Dr. Burkenstock's Protocol was so different than the other doctors I have seen. She listened to me, and together, we created a unique action plan. I love her method of blending Eastern and Western medicine philosophies," Jennifer said. "She didn't just treat my symptoms; she looked for the root causes of my issues and fixed them."

Within a few months, Jennifer reported feeling like a new person. "I have energy again. I'm sleeping better than I have in years. And that brain fog? Nonexistent! I feel sharp and focused. I didn't realize how much I'd missed out on until I started feeling better."

## Jennifer's Treatment Plan

I found Jennifer to have estradiol, estriol, and DHEA deficiencies and a sluggish thyroid. In addition, her triglycerides were very high, signifying a probable Omega-3 deficiency. Her morning cortisol was consistently low, suggesting adrenal fatigue. I initiated our DHEA, Adrenal Balance, Omega Pure fish oil supplements, and bioidentical natural hormones. I recommended that she stop using soy products (soy sauce, soybeans, tofu, and edamame) as soy aggravates thyroid and hormone function. I added Brazil nuts to her diet, which are rich in selenium to support the thyroid. These steps promote her natural thyroid hormone production.

These stories are just a tiny sample of the daily transformations in my practice. They illustrate the power of a personalized, holistic approach to women's health. Whether it's balancing hormones, losing weight, improving skin health, or boosting overall vitality, the key is to look at the whole person and address underlying imbalances.

---

**Life isn't about finding yourself.**
**Life is about creating yourself.**
~George Bernard Shaw

---

Join me, Dr. B., on the path to creating your best self.

Ready to transform your life!
Scan or Call now to schedule a consult with Dr. Burkenstock.

985-727-7676

## YOU ARE SO WORTH IT!...

As we conclude this book, I want to emphasize that these transformations are possible for you, too. It's never too late to champion your health and start living your best, gorgeous life. Remember, you are unique, and your approach to a fabulous life should be, too.

You are so worth investing in your health and well-being. You deserve to feel vibrant, confident, lovely, and healthy at every stage of life. This book has given you my knowledge and inspiration to start and continue your wellness journey.

Just when the caterpillar thought the world was over, **SHE** became a butterfly!

*~Proverb*

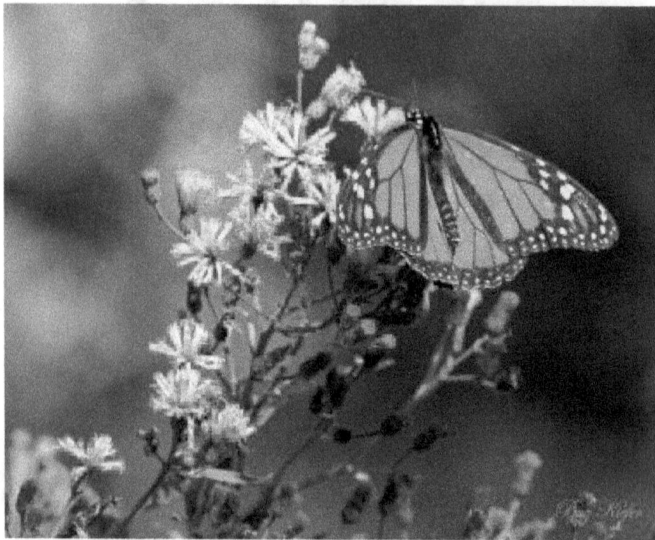

Thank you for joining me on this journey through women's health and wellness. Here's to living your best life at any age because... *You Are So Worth It! Cheers!*

# About the Author

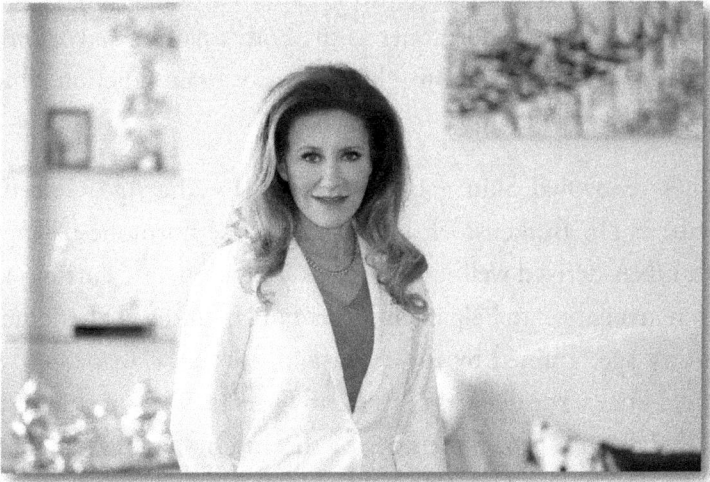

Dr. Kelly Gilthorpe Burkenstock, M.D., M.B.A.

Dr. Burkenstock is a national speaker, educator, and recognized expert in menopause and hormone optimization. She is also the founder of Skin • Body • Health – The Age Gracefully Institute.

Everything Dr. Kelly G. Burkenstock does reflects her conviction that every client deserves the very best. A national leader in menopause care and hormone optimization, she helps women and men navigate midlife transitions with science-backed therapies that restore energy, mood, skin vitality, and quality of life.

Dr. Burkenstock holds a Fellowship in Anti-Aging and Regenerative Medicine, serves on the Advisory Board of The Menopause Association (MenopauseAssociation.org), is a regular contributor on RedefiningMenopause.com, and is a Constituent of the International Society for Sexual Medicine (ISSM) as well as a long-standing member of the Sexual Medicine Society of North America (SMSNA). She has spent decades mastering advanced strategies for bioidentical hormone therapy, perimenopause and fertility support, and preventive hormone-driven health care. Her approach treats hormones as the body's natural *"orchestra"*—balancing each note to protect bone density, brain function, libido, skin, and overall vitality.

At her renowned Skin • Body • Health – The Age Gracefully Institute, Dr. Burkenstock integrates precise hormone balancing with DNA-derived wellness solutions, nutrition, and cutting-edge skin rejuvenation to help clients look radiant and feel phenomenal at every age. Trained by top experts in Europe, Canada, and the United States, she delivers consistently natural, elegant skin results and has been a proud member of the International Academy of Cosmetic Dermatology (IACD) for over 15 years.

Her New Orleans roots infuse her care with charisma, warmth, and a dash of spice—qualities that make clients feel both confident and supported. Beyond her clinical work, she champions women's health education and serves causes close to her heart, including the Safe Harbor Domestic Violence Foundation, the American Heart Association's Go Red movement, and breast-cancer research.

Guided by the belief that *"we rise by lifting others,"* Dr. Burkenstock empowers every individual to embrace balanced hormones, graceful aging, and vibrant health—at any stage of life.

www.ingramcontent.com/pod-product-compliance
Lightning Source LLC
Chambersburg PA
CBHW060859280326
41934CB00007B/1119